Abdominal Surgery -
A Brief Overview

*Edited by Ahmad Zaghal
and Arwa El Rifai*

Published in London, United Kingdom

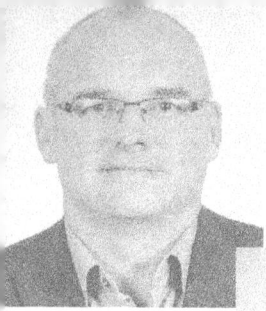
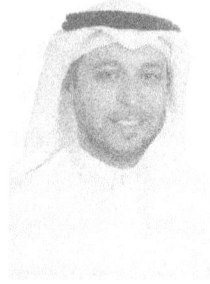
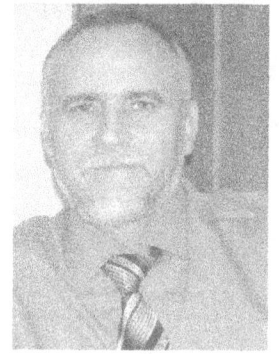
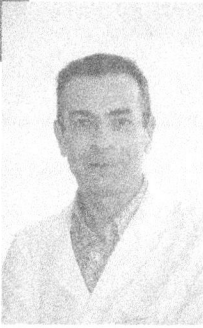
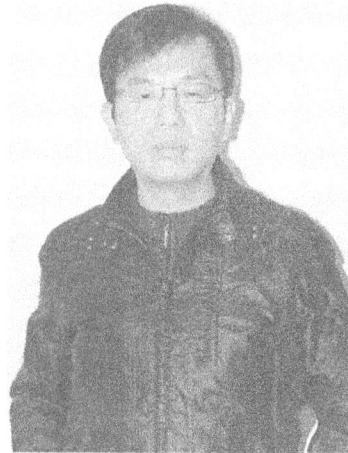
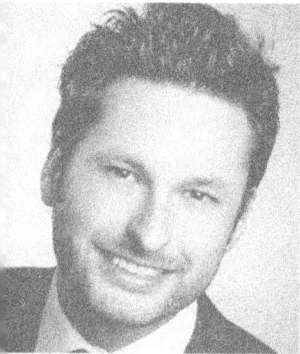
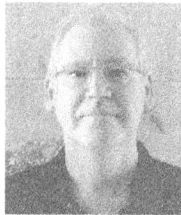

IntechOpen

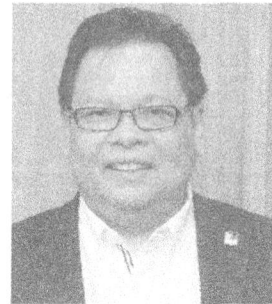
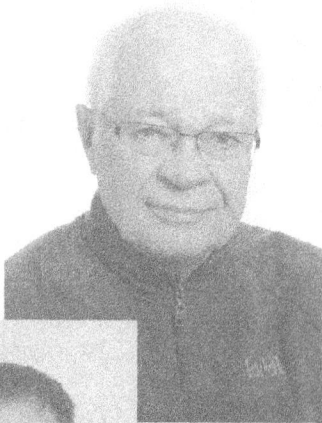
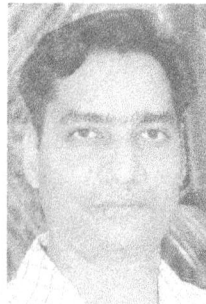
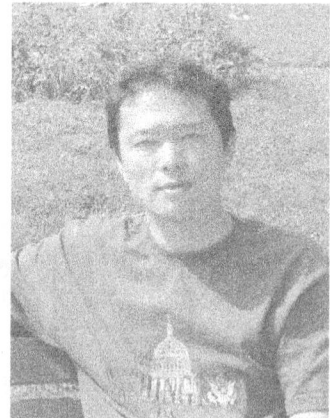
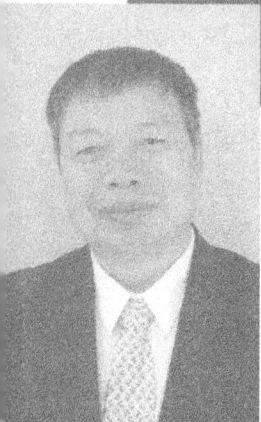
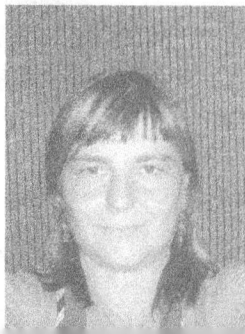

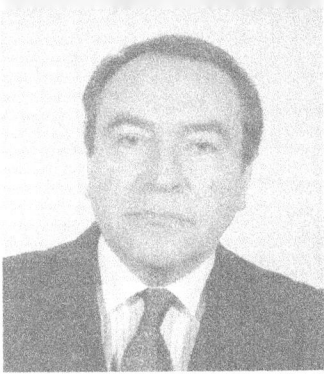

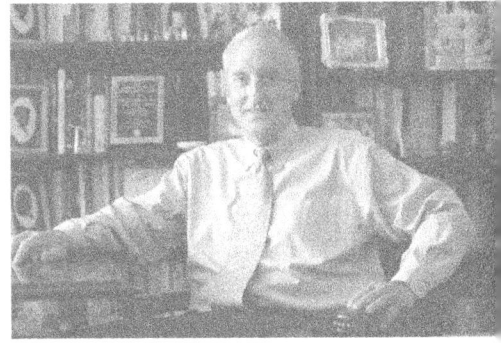

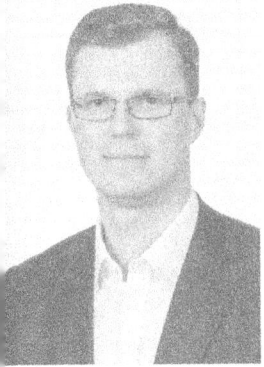

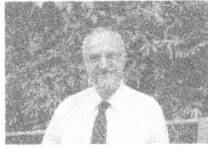

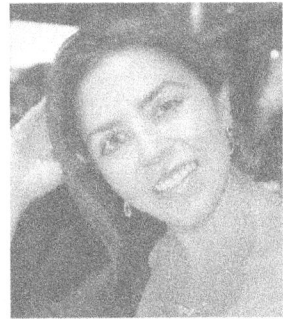

Supporting open minds since 2005

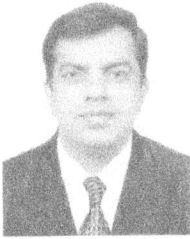

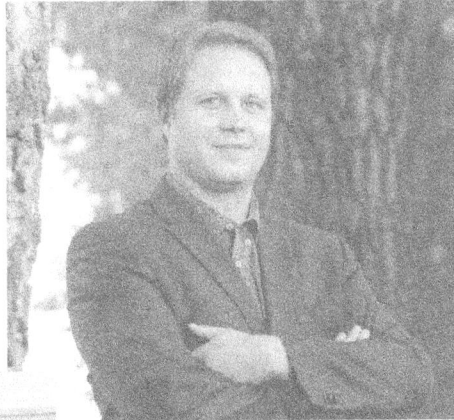

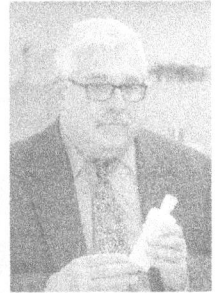

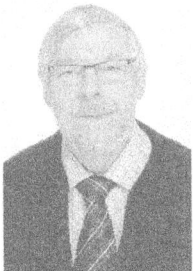

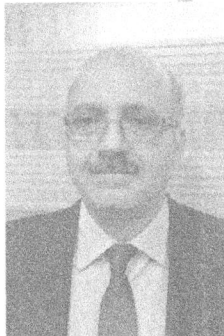

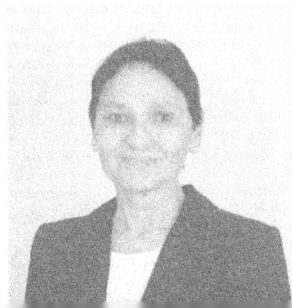

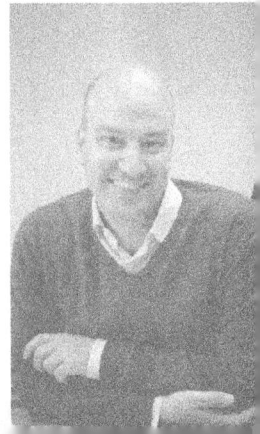

Abdominal Surgery - A Brief Overview
http://dx.doi.org/10.5772/intechopen.91538
Edited by Ahmad Zaghal and Arwa El Rifai

Contributors
Andrea Sanna, Luca Felicioni, Alpha Oumar Toure, Ousmane Thiam, Mohamadou Lamine Gueye, Mamadou Seck, Leen jamel Doya, Ali Ibrahim, Stelian Stefanita Mogoanta, Carmen Aurelia Mogoanta, Stefan Paitici, Ahmad Zaghal, Arwa El Rifai, Arwa El-Rifai

Notice
Statements and opinions expressed in the chapters are these of the individual contributors and not necessarily those of the editors or publisher. No responsibility is accepted for the accuracy of information contained in the published chapters. The publisher assumes no responsibility for any damage or injury to persons or property arising out of the use of any materials, instructions, methods or ideas contained in the book.

First published in London, United Kingdom, 2021 by IntechOpen
IntechOpen is the global imprint of INTECHOPEN LIMITED, registered in England and Wales, registration number: 11086078, 5 Princes Gate Court, London, SW7 2QJ, United Kingdom
Printed in Croatia

British Library Cataloguing-in-Publication Data
A catalogue record for this book is available from the British Library

Additional hard and PDF copies can be obtained from orders@intechopen.com

Abdominal Surgery - A Brief Overview
Edited by Ahmad Zaghal and Arwa El Rifai
p. cm.
Print ISBN 978-1-83968-671-9
Online ISBN 978-1-83968-672-6
eBook (PDF) ISBN 978-1-83968-673-3

We are IntechOpen,
the world's leading publisher of
Open Access books
Built by scientists, for scientists

5,400+
Open access books available

133,000+
International authors and editors

160M+
Downloads

Our authors are among the

156
Countries delivered to

Top 1%
most cited scientists

12.2%
Contributors from top 500 universities

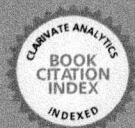

Interested in publishing with us?
Contact book.department@intechopen.com

Numbers displayed above are based on latest data collected.
For more information visit www.intechopen.com

Meet the editors

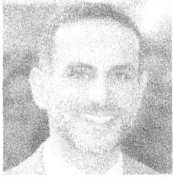

Ahmad Zaghal, MD, FEBPS, FHEA, graduated from the general surgery-residency program at The American University of Beirut-Medical Center (AUBMC), Lebanon, in 2012. He then completed a two-year fellowship in Pediatric Surgery at the University of Iowa-Hospitals and Clinics, USA. Then he joined Chelsea and Westminster Hospital, UK, for another year of fellowship in pediatric surgery. Dr. Zaghal is board certified by the European Board of Pediatric Surgery. Dr. Zaghal has been a pediatric surgeon and assistant professor of surgery at AUBMC since 2017. He has special interests in minimally invasive and neonatal surgery, and medical education. He is a fellow of the Higher Education Academy. Dr. Zaghal has published several articles in peer-reviewed journals and authored several chapters in general and pediatric surgery.

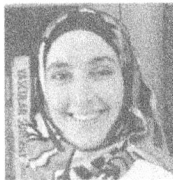

Dr. Arwa El Rifai graduated from the Faculty of Medicine, American University of Beirut (AUB), in 2015, after which she completed her training in the Department of General Surgery at the AUB Medical Center. After graduation, Dr. El Rifai joined the Clemenceau Medical Center as a surgical fellow. Dr. El Rifai is currently serving as a medical advisor for Johnson and Johnson in the Middle East. Her interest is in colorectal and oncology surgery with a focus on innovation, technology, and shaping healthcare and policy in the region.

Contents

Preface

Abdominal surgery is at the heart of general and pediatric surgical practice. It includes a broad spectrum of surgical procedures such as appendectomy, cholecystectomy, resection of abdominal tumors, and procedures for gastro-esophageal reflux disease, among many other surgeries. Indications, preoperative and postoperative patient care, and approaches and techniques involved with abdominal surgeries have been a subject of clinical research for a long time with many questions remaining unanswered.

This book is for junior surgeons in practice, surgical trainees, medical and nursing students, as well as all healthcare practitioners involved with the care of patients undergoing abdominal surgeries. It provides readers with a comprehensive overview of the theoretical and practical knowledge necessary for healthcare providers to look after their patients who are planning to or have already undergone an abdominal surgical procedure. This book outlines common indications of abdominal procedures in both adults and children and discusses important technical aspects of abdominal surgeries such as laparoscopic versus open approaches, incision types, fascial closure techniques, and the use of peritoneal drains. This is in addition to information on state-of-the-art preoperative preparation and postoperative patient care guidelines, and a discussion of potential complications of abdominal surgeries.

Ahmad Zaghal, MD, FEBPS, FHEA and Arwa El Rifai, MD
Department of Surgery,
American University of Beirut Medical Center,
Beirut, Lebanon

Chapter 1

Introductory Chapter: Abdominal Surgeries

Arwa El-Rifai and Ahmad Zaghal

1. Historical background

Over the past centuries, knowledge about abdominal pathologies and management transformed gradually into the field we know today. The elucidation of the multiplicity of diseases underlying Hippocrates "ileus" came after the tremendous efforts, successes and often failures of the surgical forefathers. Far from being a comprehensive timeline, from the coining of "peritonitis" to the description of appendicitis to the successful treatment of an appendiceal abscess was a journey that took nearly a hundred years. However, the breakthrough of anesthesia and asepsis in the 1840s and 1870s respectively brought about surgical innovation and advancement at unprecedented pace [1].

2. Examples of abdominal surgeries

Abdominal surgeries constitute a heterogeneous group of procedures that constitute the core of the general and pediatric surgical practice as well as a multitude of surgical training programs. This includes a long list of operations that are performed on elective and emergency basis. Classic examples include, but not limited to, the resection of inflamed gastrointestinal organs such as appendectomy for acute appendicitis and cholecystectomy for acute cholecystitis, operations for complicated inflammatory bowel diseases such as Crohn's disease and ulcerative colitis, bariatric operations such as sleeve gastric resections and gastric bypass, tumor resections such as Whipple procedure for pancreatic malignancies, and bowel resections for colon cancer. Laparotomies also allow repair of diaphragmatic hernias both congenital and acquired, vascular procedures such as emergency and elective repair of abdominal aortic aneurysms. Liver procedures are also an important example of abdominal procedures such as liver resections for malignant conditions of the liver. Other indications include repair of the abdominal wall and inguinal hernias, gastro-esophageal reflux, hiatal hernias, abdominal trauma, and bowel obstruction among others. Moreover, urologists and gynecologists also perform abdominal surgeries for a wide variety of indications including and not limited to uterine and ovarian resections for a variety of malignant and benign conditions, nephrectomies, urinary bladder resections and reconstructions, pyeloplasties and other procedures.

3. Minimally invasive approach

A relatively recent momentum is shifting the operative paradigm towards a minimally invasive approach. Initially with the advent of laparoscopy that re-invented the surgical technique to single port access and advanced robotic platforms. Minimally invasive approaches in abdominal surgeries reduce the postoperative recovery time and allow for an earlier return to normal life, is associated with reduced risk of wound-related infections and bowel obstruction related to adhesion formation, this is in addition to its cosmetic superiority over the classic open approach [2]. That said, the open abdominal procedure remains an important element of the general surgeons' armamentarium with its valid indications, such as in cases of hemodynamically unstable trauma patients (such as in shattered spleens and high grade liver lacerations), bowel obstruction with massive intestinal distention, and large tumors involving major abdominal vessels particularly in children such as in patients with large neuroblastoma.

4. Dilemmas in abdominal surgeries

Indications, preoperative and postoperative patient care, approaches and techniques involved with abdominal surgeries have been a subject of clinical research for a long time; some questions have been answered with relatively high confidence based on well-designed clinical and non-clinical trials while many other questions remain unanswered and subject to debate. Examples of commonly discussed dilemmas include the following:

1. What is the ideal prepping solution for disinfecting the abdominal skin before surgeries? Betadine-based or chlorhexidine-based?

2. What is the best type of and technique for bowel-to-bowel anastomosis?

3. Which is better: hand-sewn or stapled anastomosis?

4. Which type of suture material is ideal for bowel anastomosis, fascial and abdominal wall closure?

5. How can the risk of post-operative superficial and deep wound infection complications be reduced?

6. What is the role of bowel preparation before surgeries involving the colon and rectum? Mechanical preparation versus chemical preparation.

7. When is non-operative management indicated versus surgical explorations in specific disease processes?

5. Focus and content

The primary focus of this book is to present a brief and basic overview on abdominal surgeries, both theoretical knowledge and practical tips and clues. Our target audiences are junior general and pediatric surgeons in practice, obstetricians and gynecologists, urologists, surgical and medical residents and fellows, operating room and surgical ward nurses, medical and nursing students, and all other healthcare providers involved with the care of patients undergoing abdominal procedures of any type. The book tackles common indications for surgeries of the abdomen across all age groups, as well some important technical considerations such as minimally invasive approaches, wound closure and bowel anastomosis techniques, and the indications, pros and cons of the utilization of peritoneal drains after abdominal surgeries. In addition, this book reviews the up-to-date perioperative care guidelines and recommendations. That said, this book is not intended to be a comprehensive reference for all the abdominal surgical pathologies and details of the surgical techniques.

6. Conclusion

We hope that this book will provide the readers with a general flavor and basic information around the different types, indications, and potential complications of abdominal surgeries as well as the optimal care of patients undergoing abdominal procedures.

Author details

Arwa El-Rifai and Ahmad Zaghal*
Department of Surgery, American University of Beirut-Medical Center,
Beirut, Lebanon

*Address all correspondence to: az22@aub.edu.lb

IntechOpen

References

[1] Ellis H. (2010) A Brief History of Emergency Abdominal Surgery. In: Schein M., Rogers P., Assalia A. (eds) Schein's Common Sense Emergency Abdominal Surgery. Springer, Berlin, Heidelberg. https://doi.org/10.1007/978-3-540-74821-2_2

[2] Buia, A., Stockhausen, F., & Hanisch, E. (2015). Laparoscopic surgery: A qualified systematic review. World journal of methodology, 5(4), 238-254. https://doi.org/10.5662/wjm.v5.i4.238

Chapter 2

Paraumbilical/Umbilical Hernia

Andrea Sanna and Luca Felicioni

Abstract

Umbilical hernia is a common pathology that occurs in around 2% of the population. About 10% of abdominal hernias are umbilical hernias and umbilical hernia repair is among the most commonly performed surgeries in adults. The diagnosis is straightforward when tissues or organs such as the omentum or a bowel segment bulge out through an opening in the muscles of the abdominal wall in the umbilical region. The treatment options for umbilical hernia include non-operative and operative management strategies via open or minimally invasive techniques. This chapter provides a comprehensive review of umbilical hernias in adults.

Keywords: hernias, abdominal hernia, umbilical hernia, mesh, surgery

1. Introduction

Hernias constitute a broad spectrum of a well-known clinical entity and run throughout the whole history of humankind. One of the first illustrations that describe an umbilical hernia (UH) is seen in a Phoenician terracotta sculpture from the 4th–5th century B.C. Abdominal hernias are defined as a protrusion of structures through a defect of the abdominal wall that normally contains it. An umbilical hernia is a primary ventral hernia with the defect located in the midline at-or within 3 cm around the umbilicus. [1, 2] This is a common type of hernia in the adult population and is exceeded only by the inguinal hernia. Approximately up to 166,000 primary umbilical hernia repairs are performed annually in the United States. [3]

2. Epidemiology

It was estimated that about 2% of adult population have an umbilical hernia that is clinically demonstrable [1–5]. The results of a study performed by a radiologist on the ultrasound examination of the anterior abdominal wall examination wall done, for reasons other than hernia, showed that asymptomatic UH may be present with an incidence of 25% in females and 23% in males. [4, 5] The incidence rate of UH varies substantially with age and gender. The age-specific prevalence is typically higher for men (61–70 years), compared to women (31–40 years); adipose deposition differs between men and women, this may contribute to the gender differences in the development of UH. Furthermore, the overall numbers of UH repairs are higher in men than in women. [4–8]

3. Etiology and pathophysiology

There are several risk factors for the development of umbilical/paraumbilical hernia, some are congenital and others are acquired (90% of cases). (**Figure 1**). [1–3, 8, 9] Congenital UH is related to an incomplete closure of the umbilical ring, which usually, closes spontaneously within three to five years after birth; in cases of umbilical hernia development, the ring does not close and the muscles which should unite during development fail to form a strong union. A large portion of umbilical hernias labeled as "acquired hernias" because they are diagnosed in adulthood, knowing that some of these may be present from birth but have gone undetected. Despite many studies involving UH, there is lack of data on its development; commonly documented causes for acquired UH include the following: connective tissue disorder (lower type I collagen), overweight, pregnancy (frequent or multiple gestation pregnancies), obesity, ascites, cirrhosis, rectus diastase, peritoneal dialysis, large abdominal tumor, and trisomy 21 syndrome. [8, 9] All conditions that may cause an increase in the intra-abdominal pressure that results in stretching of the abdominal muscles and separate muscle bundles which weaken the fascial layer strength and favor the occurrence of UH. [1, 2, 8, 9] Another factor that has been evaluated over the past decade is the rising rates of obesity in adolescents and adult population. Sports hernia is one particular form of this disease addressed in athletes. Despite the higher prevalence of inguinal hernias in athletes, the anatomical and biomechanical considerations of the central abdominal wall theoretically makes the umbilical are at risk for hernia formation in this group of individuals. That may be due to disproportionate pull of abdominal rectus muscles as the proposed mechanism for creation of inguinal hernias in athletes. [7–9]

In adults, the abdominal wall usually has sufficient strength to resist rising abdominal pressure to prevent herniation of intra-abdominal contents. In certain abdominal wall weakening conditions, such as chronic abdominal distension the rising pressure from within may be responsible for the occurrence of UH. [10]

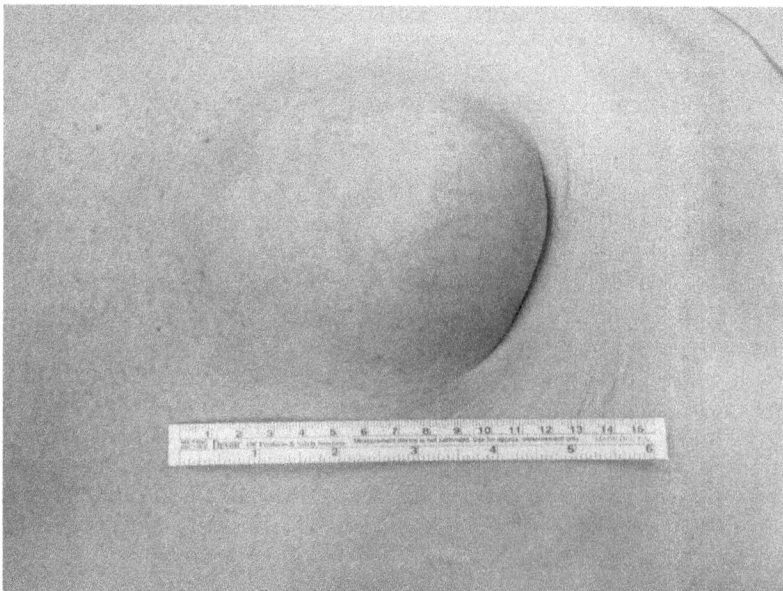

Figure 1.
Umbilical hernia stranguled.

Hernia development is more common in pregnancy due to two main components, hormonally induced increased laxity of the pelvic ligaments and high abdominal pressure. It is also more common in the elderly due to degenerative weakness of muscles and fibrous tissue. [1, 2, 7, 8]

4. Clinical history and presentation

The presentation of UH is variable, from asymptomatic to requiring emergency surgery (4% after 5 years). [1, 2, 4, 8] Small-size hernia with incarcerated omentum could produce intermittent or constant pain, sometimes associated with general symptoms. Larger hernias may be asymptomatic. Patients often present with mild symptoms, some degree of discomfort usually appears first. UH typically, presents with protrusion or bulging under the skin at the umbilical ring, one should determine whether the hernia reduces spontaneously or needs to be reduced manually. Progressively, the hernia (fascial) defect enlarges and in most cases becomes tender or irreducible with time. Severe pain should alert the surgeon to a high risk of strangulation: compromised blood supply to herniated tissues/organs. This is a serious complication with signs of skin color changes and, intestinal obstruction if the sac contains a loop of small bowel (**Figure 1**). It is important to remember that UH can lead to complications many of which can be fatal if not properly treated. Strangulation can occur in irreducible, also known as incarcerated hernias, and can lead to peritonitis, septic shock and a rapid deterioration in the patient's condition. Some reports show that older age, female gender, umbilical hernia defects between 2 and 7 cm are potential risk factors for the development of acute complications. [1, 2, 7, 9]

The European Hernia Society and Americas Hernia Society (EHS and AHS) classification for umbilical/epigastric hernia is a clinically relevant system based on defect diameter (**Table 1**). [8]

Primary Umbilical Hernia size	Dimension
Small	1.1 cm
Medium	More than 1 cm up to 4 cm
Large	Over 4 cm

Table 1.
The European and Americas hernia society classification for umbilical/epigastric.

5. Diagnosis and investigations

Umbilical hernia is usually diagnosed by inspection and palpation with the patient lying down and standing, as this will usually make the hernia bulge more apparent and demonstrable. The patient is asked to cough or make a Valsalva's maneuver, this can cause an occult hernia to be more evident. It is important to estimate both the fascial defect size and hernia content. Careful examination of the entire abdominal wall is crucial in order to evaluate for hernia complications or the presence of multiple defects. Skin must be evaluated, the appearance of bruises suggests venous engorgement of the hernia contents; this may be due to underlying complications such as incarceration or strangulation. Local and generalized abdominal pain, irreducible hernia, fever, leucocytosis and signs of bowel obstruction are signs that warrant immediate attention and management as they may potentially be related to significant complications.

When a patient has symptoms but no hernia demonstrated on meticulous and detailed physical exam, or there is clinical uncertainty, imaging may be helpful to establish the diagnosis. In these patients, abdominal ultrasound and/or computed tomography are very useful in establishing the diagnosis as well as preoperatively planning, for instance, they can influence surgical decision making in terms of choosing open versus laparoscopic approaches [3].

6. Management

There are two main treatment options for patients with umbilical hernia, non-operative management and surgical repair. Non-operative management can be divided into three categories:

1. Non-operative management except for acute presentations suitable for high-risk patients.

2. Initial non-operative management: in symptomatic or patients who desire to have the hernia repaired but have modifiable risk factors such as smoking, uncontrolled diabetes, BMI > 30 Kg/m^2).

3. Watchful waiting and "wait for symptoms to appear": suitable in patients with acceptable surgical risks but have few hernia symptoms or signs [1, 2, 4, 7–9, 11].

Outcomes of patients treated non-operatively and the risk of delayed acute presentation are unclear. However data from a retrospective study showed that within 5 years of follow-up 4% of cases underwent surgical procedures in emergency settings. Little is known about the results of watchful waiting approach in patients with UH but this strategy seems safe.

The common risks of non-operative management include increasing discomfort or pain (worsening during coughing and defecation), increasing hernia size, skin complications, constipation due to worsening abdominal function and acute presentations such as sharp pain and irreducibility.

Typically, adult symptomatic umbilical hernias need to be fixed to reduce the potential risk of complications. Umbilical hernia repair can be achieved with either sutured or mesh repair. The latest guidelines by SAGE and EHS-AHS (European Hernia Society-American Hernia Society) recommended the mesh usage in order to reduce hernia recurrences. Sutured repair can be considered for small-size hernia defects of less than one cm [9].

Umbilical hernia repair can be achieved either via an open procedure or minimally invasive surgery as laparoscopic or robotic technique.

6.1 Open umbilical hernia repair, suture alone

Mayo technique has been considered for many years to be the standard technique for primary umbilical hernia repair. This technique, described in 1901, involves a fascial closure using two suture lines: some interrupted permanent sutures and some running absorbable sutures; the author found that the transverse direction of closure may be advantageous. [11] The recurrence rates with this technique has remained high over time. The modified technique used today is a simple defect closure with a single line of sutures. It is recommend to use non-absorbable sutures in order to reduce hernia recurrence (low level of evidence). [8] It is important to remember that sutured repair of primary small umbilical hernia (<1 cm) with the presence of muscles diastasis is a significant risk factor for recurrence, hence prosthetic reinforcement, using a mesh, for clean cases is recommended. [12]

6.2 Open umbilical hernia mesh repair

An infra-umbilical incision is usually used (transverse and vertical incision shave similar outcomes) and then the umbilical stalk is dissected. The hernia sac is dissected down to the fascia. Reduction of hernia sac and its content into abdominal cavity is done. Fascial edges should be refurbished by incising at least 2 mm margins from the umbilical ring. Gentle blunt dissection to the posterior rectus sheath is done to prepare the posterior field. A space of 5 cm in all directions should be developed. The mesh generally can be placed in either the sublay position (retrorectus space) or the underlay pre-peritoneal position. Moreover, there are commercially available umbilical hernia patches with mesh coated by tissue-separating layer designed to allow for intra-peritoneal mesh placement. The defect can be closed with absorbable or non-absorbable sutures [13, 14]. The skin closure is done with material based on the surgeon's preferences.

6.3 MIS: Intraperitonial Onlay mesh (IPOM)

To be able to perform the IPOM repair, preparation of the needed laparoscopic instruments is imperative. These include: camera port, one 11 mm blunt trocar, one 5 mm trocar, 30°endoscope, bipolar coagulation clamp, monopolar coagulation scissor. The patient is placed in the supine position with bilateral arms tucked to the sides on a flexed table. The monitor is placed in front of the surgeon. Pneumoperitoneum is then established with the surgeon's preferred technique (Verres needle, open approach, optically trocar). A 12 mmHg CO_2 pressure creates the working space. Once a good working space is established, either an 11 or 5-mm trocars are placed on the left lateral side. The hernia ring is dissected with reduction of the contents and the hernia sac. Usually peritoneal fat and falciform ligament are dissected to expose the fascia. This is important in order to improve mesh fixation which is done using tacs to anchor and prevent the mesh from sliding [15]. Hernia defect closure is a good practice and can be performed using absorbable barbed sutures either laparoscopically or using Reverdin needle techniques, based on surgeon's preferences, may be used. Based on the published literature, it is reasonable to cover the hernia defect with 3–5 cm mesh overlap to avoid hernia recurrences (primary UH repair open or MIS technique). The coated mesh is then secured to the abdominal wall using double crown absorbable or non-absorbable. [16–20] The procedure may be performed either laparoscopically or robotically with some variations pertaining to docking and positioning. [20]

6.4 MIS: retro-rectus repair (Rives-Stoppa)

Several advances brought about by the prosthetics mesh industry, allowed for an effective intraperitoneal mesh placement for UH repair. However, safety problems have been raised and were reported in some cases series. In these series, late complication that emerged included adhesions, fistula formation, mesh migrations, and further damage to the abdominal viscera. In an attempt to reduce the incidence of these complications many authors proposed the placement of the prosthesis between the recto-muscle and posterior rectus fascia (retro-muscular) or between the posterior rectus sheath and the peritoneum when possible.

Several methods have been suggested by different authors to achieve the retro-muscle or preperitoneal mesh placement. These techniques include theeTEP (enhanched-view Totally Extra-Peritoneal), MILOS (Minimally Invasive Less Open Sublay), Emilos, (Endoscopic/MILOS), Costa "the Brazilian technique", TARUP (Robotic Transabdominal Retromuscular Umbilical Prosthetic) [15–22]. Moreover, some of these surgical techniques can be performed using minimally invasive approaches as posterior component separation technique (advancement of rectus-muscle), to allows reconstruction of large abdominal wall defects.

6.5 MIS: enhanced-view totally extraperitoneal (eTEP) retromuscular hernia repair

We describe eTEP technique popularized by Dr. Jorge Daes in 2012 and Belyansky in 2017 (used in inguinal hernia repair and in incisional ventral hernia repair), this technique enlarges the surgical field in comparison with the conventional TEP procedure, this approach can be performed either laparoscopically or robotically. Equipment for laparoscopic instrumentation, as we have previously described, included: camera port, one 12 mm blunt trocar, one 5 mm trocars (all with balloon), 30° endoscope, bipolar coagulation clamp, monopolar coagulation scissor, articulating radio frequency device [17, 22]. The patient is placed supine with bilateral arms tucked by the sides.

Foley catheter is placed in all cases. Operating room table is flexed as indicated by Belyansky. [16] The monitor is placed in front of the surgeon. The key elements of port placement depend on defect extension, lower midline umbilical hernia defects or upside midline umbilical hernia defect (**Figures 2, 3**). [16–21] The eTEP

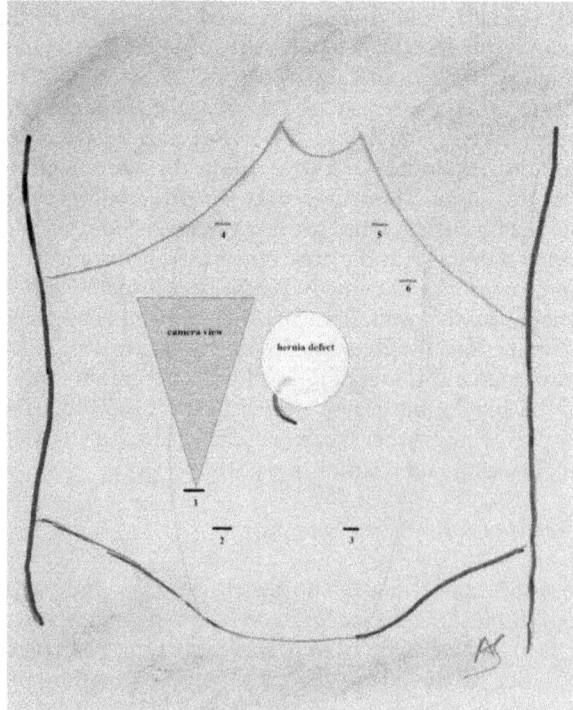

Figure 2.
Port position for upper side defects (black line; red line trocars additional).

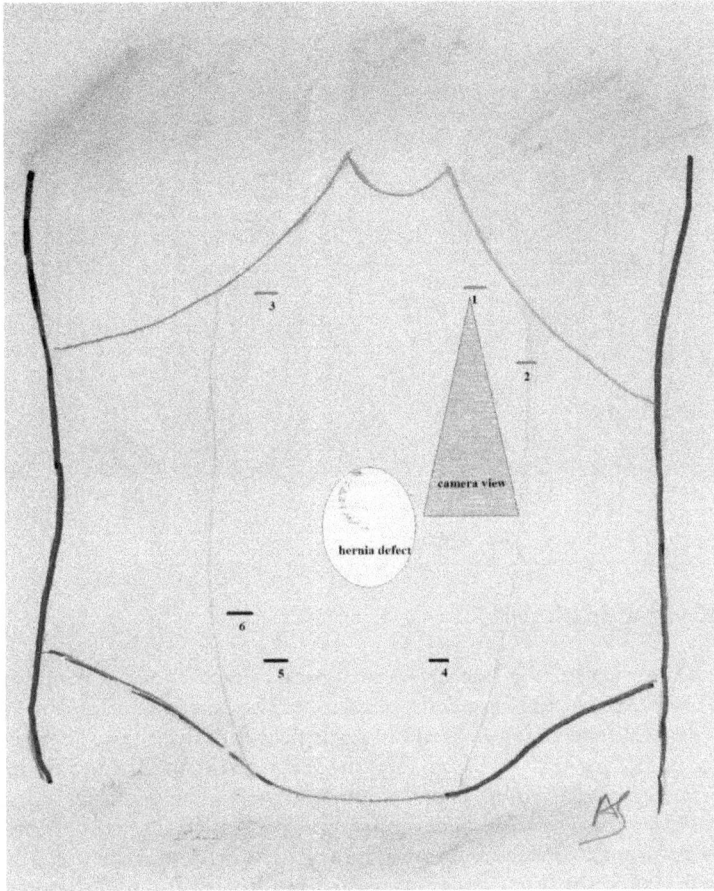

Figure 3.
Port position for lover side defects (red line; black line trocars aditional).

umbilical hernia repair technique begins with a one side retro-rectus dissection. The first incision is indicated with by the camera view as in **Figures 2, 3**. The anterior rectus sheath is incised. The rectus muscle fibers are opened and working space is created with a balloon dissector. Carbone dioxide is used as in laparoscopic techniques to establish pneumoperitoneum. A 6–8 mmHg CO2 pressure is set inside the working space. Dissection of one retro-rectus space is made with energy source (bipolar articulating tissue sealer or radio frequency device). Other trocars are placed as described in **Figures 2, 3**. Extra trocars can be placed if deemed necessary. Then crossing over to the contralateral retrorectus space, the two space are joined. Gentle dissection of the tissue is performed without violating the perito-neum. Then the, right posterior sheath is dissected to achieve the right retro-rectus space. Dissection of right retro-rectus space is made and the right and left posterior sheath are divide both until arcuate line (**Figure 4**). Laterally the dissection is limited by the linea semilunaris. The hernia ring is dissected with reduction of the contents and hernia sac. Posterior defect is closed using 2–0 absorbable barbed sutures. The hernia defect is closed too with number 0 absorbable barbed suture. Mesh is positioned to cover umbilical hernia defect with 5 cm of overlap. The mesh is secured with cyanoacrylate.

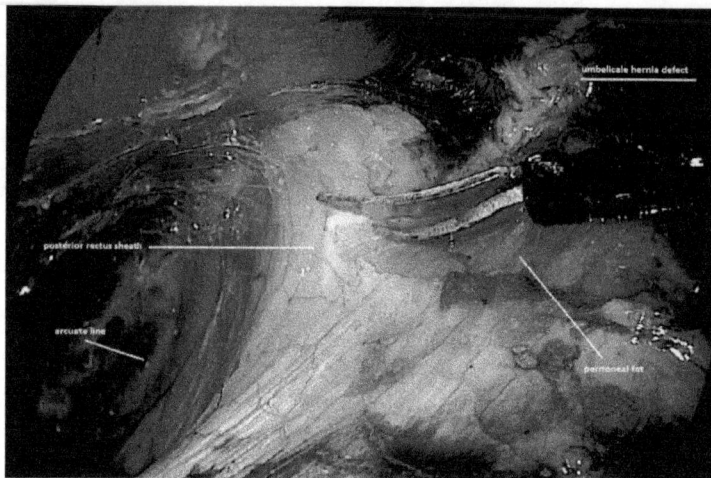

Figure 4.
Left posterior rectus sheath is incised from cephalad to caudal direction.

7. Surgical complications

Umbilical hernia repair is associated with good outcomes and a lower rates of hernias recurrences and overall complications. The hernia size and the fascial defect are important risk factors predicting surgical complications. There is still a spectrum of complications within each of these categories including minor wound separation and complete wound separation both of which would be categorized as wound dehiscence. The leading complications include wound complications (seroma, haematoma, infections), bowel injury and hernia recurrences. [2, 7]. The disadvantage of synthetic mesh placement must be considered; however, no significant differences in complication rates when comparing mesh to suture repair.

Recent studies have shown lower rate of mesh complications. [8] Mesh infection complicates in most cases open ventral hernia repairs than laparoscopic repairs. Mesh erosion into the gastro-intestinal tract is published and likely an underreported late complication of mesh placement particularly the intra-peritoneal mesh position which has been associated with erosion and the development of late fistula.

8. Conclusions

Since the original description by Mayo in 1901, a wide variety of options became available for the repair of umbilical hernias, in order to reduce surgical morbidity and improve the patient's quality of life. Umbilical hernia is a disease process that requires the general surgeon to have a wide armamentarium of repair techniques. An understanding of anatomy is key for tailored treatment. Utilization of advanced techniques requires careful patient selection, knowledge of abdominal wall anatomy and technical details in order to reduce the need for reoperations. Several of these innovations, including either minimally invasive techniques and the uses of different types and positions of meshes to be used in reinforcement. Despite this, it is clear that mesh repair of incisional and inguinal hernias reduces recurrence rates, the impact of mesh for umbilical hernia repair remains a subject of debate. To date, some prospective randomized controlled trials have addressed this question. These studies found lower recurrence rates after mesh versus primary suture repair, without a significant increase in the risk of wound-related infectious complications. Based on current evidence, primary hernia repair remains reasonable and appropriate only for small (1 cm) umbilical hernias. As always, in abdominal wall reconstruction we believe that the specific technique for repair should be tailored to the individual patient.

Acknowledgements

The authors are grateful to Dr. B,Mantovan drafted the manuscript.

Conflict of interest

The authors: A.Sanna have no conflicts of interest or financial ties to disclose. L Felicioni has received grants from Company, for others studies (2018 BARD, 2019 GEM and AB Medica).

Author details

Andrea Sanna[1*] and Luca Felicioni[2]

1 Department of General Surgery, Ospedali Riuniti Padova Sud, Padova, Italy

2 Department of General and Robotic Surgery, Ospedale della Misericordia, Grosseto, Italy

*Address all correspondence to: and_sanna@yahoo.it

IntechOpen

References

[1] Dabbas N, Adams K, Pearson K, Royle G. Frequency of abdominal hernias: is classical teaching out of date? JRSM Short Rep.2011 Jan 19;2(1):5.

[2] Coste AH, Jaafar S, Parmely JD. Umbilical Hernia. 2020 Jul 21. In: StatPearls [Internet]. Treasure Island (FL): StatPearls Publishing; 2020 Jan–. PMID: 29083594.

[3] Bedewi MA, El-Sharkawy MS, Al Boukai AA, Al-Nakshabandi N. Prevalence of adult paraumbilical hernia. Assessment by high-resolution sonography: a hospital-based study. Hernia. 2012 Feb;16(1):59-62. doi: 10.1007/s10029-011-0863-4. Epub 2011 Jul 28. PMID: 21796449.

[4] T.J.Swope. Umbilical Hernia options. The sages manual of hernia. Springer 2019:157-172.

[5] Hope W, Cobb WS,Adrales GL, Textbook of hernia. Springer, 2017

[6] Shankar DA, Itani KMF, O'Brian WJ, Sanchez VM. Factors associated with long-term outcomes of umbilical hernia repair. Jama Surg.2017 May 01;152(5):461-466.

[7] Venclauskas L, Joukubasuskas M, Zilinskas J, Zviniene K, Kiidelis M. Long-term follow-up results umbilical hernia repair. Wideochir Inne Tech Maloinwazyjne. 2017 Dec:12(4):350-356

[8] Williams N, Rononan o'Connel P, McCaskie A. Short Pratice of surgery 27th Edition .Bailey & Love's.2017

[9] Henriksen NA, Montgomery A, Kaufmann R, Berrevoet F, East B, Fischer J, Hope W, Klassen D, Lorenz R, Renard Y, Garcia Urena MA, Simons MP; European and Americas Hernia Societies (EHS and AHS). Guidelines for treatment of umbilical and epigastric hernias from European Hernia Society and American Hernia Society. Br J Surg.020 Feb;107(3):171-190. doi: 10.1002/bjs.11489.Epub 2020 Jan 9.

[10] Farber AJ, Wilckens JH.Sports hernia: diagnosis and therapeutic approach.J Am Acad Orthop Surg. 2007;15(8):507-14. doi:10.5435/00124635-200708000-00007

[11] Kokotovic D, Sjølander H, Gögenur I, Helgstrand F. Watchful waiting as a treatment strategy for patients with a ventral hernia appears to be safe. Hernia. 2016;20(2):281-7.

[12] Mayo WJ. VI. An Operation for the Radical Cure of Umbilical Hernia. Ann Surg. 1901 Aug;34(2):276-80. doi: 10.1097/00000658-190107000-00021. PMID: 17861015; PMCID: PMC1425538.

[13] Heidi J. Miller, Yuri W. Novitsky. Ventral Hernia and Abdominal Release Procedures. Shackelford's Surgery of the Alimentary Tract, 2 Volume Set (Eighth Edition), 2019

[14] Belyansky I, Daes Köhler G, Luketina RR, Emmanuel K Sutured repair of primary small umbilical and epigastric hernias: concomitant rectus diastasis is a significant risk factor for recurrence. World J Surg 2015. 39(1):121-126

[15] Muysoms F, Vander Mijnsbrugge G, Pletinckx P, Boldo E, Jacobs I, Michiels M, Ceulemans R (2013) Randomized clinical trial of mesh fixation with "double crown" versus "sutures and tackers" in laparoscopic ventral hernia repair. Hernia 17:603-612

[16] Gonzalez AM, Romero RJ, Seetharamaiah R, Gallas M, Lamoureux J, Rabaza JR (2015) Laparoscopic ventral hernia

repair with primary closure versus no primary closure of the defect: potential benefits of the robotic technology. Int J Med Robot 11:120-125

[17] Belyansky J, Radu VG, Balasubramanian R, Reza Zahiri H, Weltz AS, Sibia US, Park A, Novitsky Y. A novel approach using the enhanced-view totally extraperitoneal (eTEP) technique for laparoscopic retromuscular hernia repair. Surg Endosc. 2018 Mar;32(3):1525-1532. doi: 10.1007/s00464-017-5840-2. Epub 2017 Sep 15.

[18] Schroeder AD, Debus ES, Reinpold WM et al Laparoscopic transperitoneal sublay mesh repair: a new technique for the cure of ventral and incisional hernias. Surg Endosc 2013.27(2):648-654

[19] W Reinpold , M Schröder , C Berger , W Stoltenberg , F Köckerling MILOS and EMILOS repair of primary umbilical and epigastric hernias Hernia. 2019 Oct;23(5):935-944. doi: 10.1007/s10029-019-02056

[20] Costa TN, Abdalla RZ, Santo MA et al Transabdominal midline reconstruction by minimally invasive surgery: technique and results. Hernia 2016. 20(2):257-265

[21] Muysoms F, Van Cleven S, Pletinckx P et al Robotic transabdominal retromuscular umbilical prosthetic hernia repair (TARUP): observational study on the operative time during the learning curve. Hernia 2018. 2(6):1101-1111

[22] Sanna A, Felicioni L, Cecconi C, Cola R.Retromuscular Mesh Repair Using Extended Totally Extraperitoneal Repair Minimal Access: Early Outcomes of an Evolving Technique—A Single Institution Experience. J Laparoendosc Adv Surg Tech A. 2020 Mar;30(3):246-250. doi: 10.1089/lap.2019.0661.

Chapter 3

Foreign Bodies Ingestion

Leen Jamel Doya and Ali Ibrahim

Abstract

Foreign body ingestion is a common problem among children especially under psychological stress. More than 110.000 ingested foreign bodies were reported in the United States, of which more than 85% occurred in the pediatric population. Ingested foreign bodies usually pass through the alimentary tract without any problem. However, they can occasionally be trapped and require endoscopic or surgical management. In the asymptomatic patient, a series of abdominal X-rays are recommended to follow up on the progress of the foreign body. When a foreign body becomes immobile in the distal bowels a high suspicion that the foreign body has become trapped must be considered and surgical management is recommended with or without signs of inflammation. Here we describe the cases scenarios of foreign bodies trapped in the gastrointestinal tract and the management options.

Keywords: Foreign bodies, surgical cases, gastrointestinal tract

1. Introduction

Foreign bodies (FBs) ingestion is a very common worldwide health problem in children between 6 months and 3 years of age (25% of them younger than 1 year) [1]. FBs ingestion affects up to 75% of children especially that infants evaluate objects by tasting and swallowing [2]. Frequent cases of FBs ingestion often occur in children with intellectual disability or those with behavioral disorders [3]. FBs ingestion generally does not cause complications and passes through the gastrointestinal tract spontaneously [4]. About 80–90% of FBs pass through the gastrointestinal (GI) tract spontaneously without complications, whereas 10–20% of them are removed endoscopically. Few children (1%) require open surgical removal secondary to complications [5]. The initial diagnosis is based on sudden onset of symptom coupled by seeing the child putting an item in his/her mouth while playing [6]. The assessment and management of FBs ingestion depends on the patient's presentation and physical examination (patient status, vital signs and airway evaluation) [7]. FBs ingestion morbidity is dependent on the type of FBs ingested; disc batteries lead to esophageal perforation and tracheoesophageal fistula formation with significant morbidity and mortality [8]. Coins and multiple magnet ingestion can require surgery to prevent secondary perforation-related attraction and necrosis of the bowel [9].

2. FBs ingestion

The risk of FBs ingestion increases in children with congenital or acquired abnormalities of the gastrointestinal tract (atresia, history of surgery) [10]. The most important issue when a foreign body enters the digestive tract is its passage through the esophagus. The esophagus has 3 physiological areas of narrowing that can potentially trap the swallowed body. 50–80% of cases of impaction of the esophagus occur at the level of the cricopharyngeal muscle above the esophagus, then the lower sphincter, and finally the site of intersection of the aorta with the esophagus [8]. FBs often pass through the digestive tract without significant problems; the estimated time of the passage through the anus is seven days [9].

3. Epidemiology and etiology of FBs ingestion

FBs ingestion is relatively serious common problem. Annually, more than 100000 cases of FBs ingestion reported each year in the United States (US); 85% occurred in pediatric population [11]. It is responsible for about (1500–3000) deaths per year in the US. There is equal incidence among boys and girls (1: 1) [12]. FBs ingestion may be accidental or deliberate. Majority of the children with FBs ingestion are healthy. Some of them have disease as strictures, achalasia, eosinophilic esophagitis, or rings [6]. The most common children FBs ingestion in US is coins, while it is different in other countries (the fish bones is most common in Asian countries). In Adolescents and adults, the most common type is food impaction [8].

4. Initial assessment

Initial assessment includes a thorough medical history should be obtained immediately to determine any medical problem and prompt physical examination should be performed [7]. FBs ingestion may be asymptomatic (10–50)% of all cases or symptomatic, depending on the location of the FBs.

In the esophagus, it may present as dysphagia, refusal of food intake, salivation, pain behind the sternum or respiratory symptoms (wheezing, stridor, frequent pneumonia, weight loss) [8].

In the stomach, it is usually asymptomatic except large FBs causes obstruction in the outlet of the stomach and appears as non-bilious vomiting and/or refusal to feed [10].

FBs in the distal parts of the gastrointestinal tract can cause right lower quadrant pain due to impaction at the level of the terminal ileum and hence mimicking acute appendicitis [11]. Neck swelling, erythema, or skin crepitus may be present on physical examination and may indicate the need for surgical consultation / intervention [8]. When the FBs is pressing on the trachea, inspiratory stridor or expiratory wheezing can be detected on the chest auscultation [9]. The most common clinical symptoms include dysphagia (37%), drooling (31%), chocking (17%). Other symptoms included: cough, abdominal pain, chest pain, stridor, vomiting, and refusal to eat [1]. FBs may lead to intestinal obstruction or perforation and present with distention or guarding on abdominal examination [10].

4.1 Radiology evaluation

Diagnosis of FBs confirmed using X-ray, barium swallow, Echography, computed tomography (CT) scan or magnetic resonance imaging (MRI). 64% of patient ingested a radiopaque object. 25–30% of FBs are not visible through X-ray, but in all cases it should be performed to look for signs of obstruction as indicated by air-fluid levels or free air indicating perforation. CT scan may be necessary to characterize the size, shape and anatomic location of the swallowed body [5].

5. Types of FBs ingestion

5.1 Coins

The most commonly ingested FBs in children are coins (80% of FBs). Approximately 30% of them, spontaneously pass through the digestive system without complications depending on its location, age of the child, and the size of the coin [7]. Coins measuring more than 23.5 mm in size are more likely to become impacted, particularly in children aged under 5 years, and coins measuring more than 25 mm in diameter are unlikely to pass through the pylorus [13]. Children with an ingested coin without any history of esophageal disease or surgery and no respiratory symptoms can be observed over 12–24 hours before performing an invasive procedure (endoscopic or surgical removal) [14].

5.2 Button batteries (BBs)

The frequency of button batteries (BBs) ingestion has increased due to their widespread use as power sources in electronic devices. Lithium batteries hold enough charge to cause harm even after they are used up [15]. The pathogenesis of BBs ingestion is dependent on the production of hydroxyl radical (OH^-) in the esophageal mucosa, causing caustic damage due to an elevated PH value in addition to thermal electrical damage [16]. PH value increases from 7 to 13 at the negative electrode of the battery 30 minutes after ingestion. Necrosis of the basal plate of the esophagus within 15 minutes of ingestion extends to the outer muscle layer within 30 minutes. The damage can last for days or weeks after the battery is removed, which can lead to death as a result of the formation of an aortic esophageal fistula after about 19 days [17]. The risk of BBs ingestion is greater in children Less than 5 years old who swallow more than 20 mm battery or multiple batteries [15]. The most important complications of BBs ingestion are necrosis, perforation, esophagotracheal fistula, cervical abscess, and stenosis of the esophagus [17]. An anterior, posterior, and lateral x-ray of the neck, chest, and abdomen should be performed which shows a double-ring sign or double halo signs in an anterior–posterior imaging (circle-within-a-circle appearance) and step-off mark in lateral appearance (characteristic two-layer appearance) [18].

5.3 Sharp or pointed foreign bodies

Sharp or pointed foreign bodies (FBs) ingestion (such as Pins, needles, bones, etc.....) is associated with high morbidity and mortality [19]. It can cause serious complications such as perforation (15–35)%, abscess formation, trachea-esophageal fistula, aortic esophageal fistula, peritonitis, and even death [20]. Less than 0.0005% of them get trapped in the appendix and require surgical management. Therefore, it is preferable to remove pointed and sharp bodies from the esophagus or stomach whenever possible to reduce the incidence of adverse events [19]. X-ray examination is necessary to diagnose radiopaque objects (as needles, pins, etc....), while radiolucent FBs such as plastic, glass, or wood cannot be identified. Therefore, an emergency endoscopy is recommended when high index of suspicion exists for ingestion of sharp FBs even with a negative X-ray [21].

5.4 Magnets

Magnet ingestion is a serious health risk associated with significant mortality and mobility. In recent years, children's ingestion of magnets has increased. The greatest risk of its ingestion when multiple magnets or a single magnet with a metallic FB has been ingested. Children may be asymptomatic or present with vomiting, cough, gagging and drooling. They may present as a result of magnet related complications [1] . It may lead to mucosal pressure necrosis, intestinal obstruction, fistula, perforation, and many other complications that necessitates surgical intervention. In addition, magnet may lead to bowel obstruction and volvulus [22]. That can lead to peritonitis, sepsis, and death.

5.5 Bezoars

A bezoar is a large ball like collections of material within the gastrointestinal system. It may be associated with pica, especially in developmentally delayed children or having psychosocial problem. Rarely, it may occur in normal children with no psychosocial issues [23]. The risk factors for the formation of a bezoar include excessive fiber consumption, chronic antacid treatment, psychiatric or developmental disorders, previous gastric surgery including vagotomy or pyloroplasty, and gastrointestinal dysmotility [24]. Bezoars are classified to phytobezoars, pharmacobezoars, trichobezoars, lactobezoars, and foreign body bezoars [25].

5.5.1 Trichobezoars or phytobezoars

It composed of bubble gum, seeds and vegetable matter. Majority in older children particularly those with psychiatric problems and young female [23].

5.5.2 Medication bezoars

It may occur in the infants treated for upper gastrointestinal bleeding or esophagitis with intragastric or frequent oral administration of aluminum hydroxide [25].

It has usually nonspecific clinical manifestations that mimic many gastrointestinal diseases [23]. Patients may present with abdominal pain, nausea, vomiting, anorexia, weight loss, intestinal bleeding from pressure ulcer necrosis, or intestinal obstruction. The most common site of bezoar is the stomach; however, It may be found in the esophagus or any site along the gastrointestinal system [24].

6. Management

There are many factors to consider when determining how to decrease the foreign bodies ingestion, especially in the extremely young. Certain object characteristics such as size, shape, and material must keep away from children. Education for parents should continue to be prioritized when possible. This can be through positions such as pediatricians, and school teachers as well as media advertisements and printed materials.

6.1 Coins

Esophageal coins must be removed within 24 hours to reduce the incidence of complications [7]. Asymptomatic children with ingested coins in the stomach should be monitored closely and the stool examined to check for the passage of the coin, and serial X-rays should be obtained every 1 or 2 weeks until the passage of the coin has been confirmed. The coin that remains in the stomach after 2–4 weeks should be endoscopically removed [11]. Patient with asymptomatic small bowel coins should be clinically observed. While children with symptoms of bowel obstruction or perforation require, surgical removal (**Figure 1**) [13].

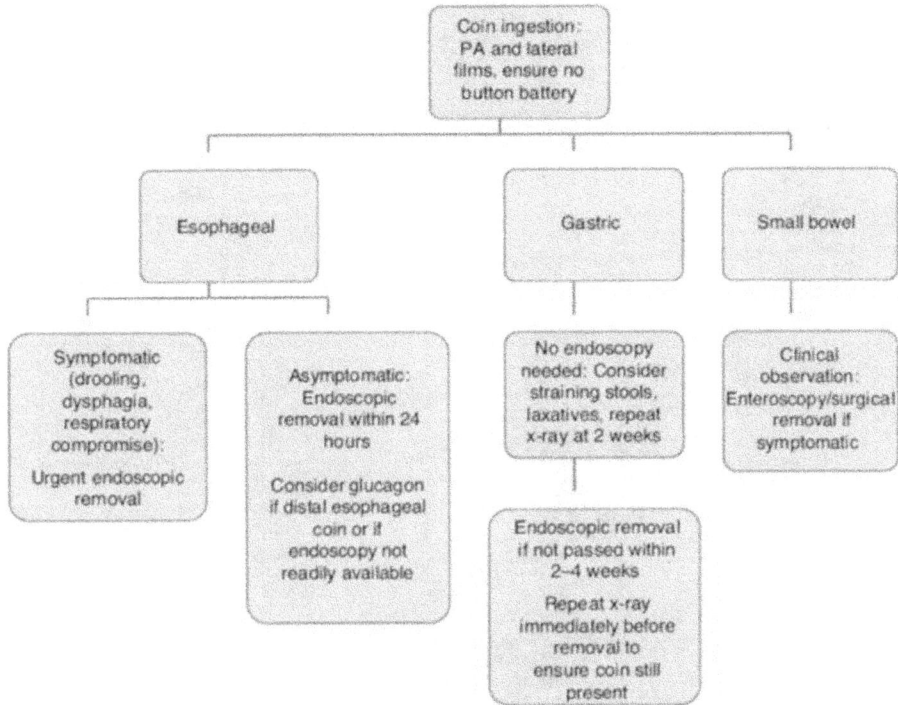

Figure 1.
Kramer's algorithm of coin ingestion.

6.2 Button batteries (BBs)

Batteries in the stomach often passed without complications. The American Society for Gastrointestinal Endoscopy (ACGE) recommendations is to extract the BBs in the stomach if the diameter is greater than 20 mm and has remained for more than 48 hours after radiological investigation [23]. The probability of the battery being expelled out of the body is 85% when it passes the duodenum within 72 hours [16]. Recent research recommends performing esophageal endoscopy in all BBs ingestion, even if they are in the stomach to evaluate the esophageal mucosa before the battery is transferred to the stomach (**Figure 2**) [26].

6.3 Sharp or pointed foreign bodies

Gastrointestinal endoscopic removal is necessary for sharp or pointed FBs, large and wide objects (more than 2.5 cm diameter in older children, more than 2 cm diameter in infants and young children), or long objects (more than 6–10 cm diameter in older children, more than 4–5 cm diameter in infants and young children) that are located in the stomach [20]. Surgical removal can be considered in symptomatic children if the FBs does not show the expected passage after 4 days or passed into the small bowel (distal to the ligament of Treitz). While asymptomatic patients should be clinically and radiographically followed-up with serial X-rays (**Figure 3**) [21].

6.4 Magnets

In asymptomatic children, an X-ray is necessary to detect whether the ingested magnets are single or multiple magnets or have a metallic part. If multiple magnets

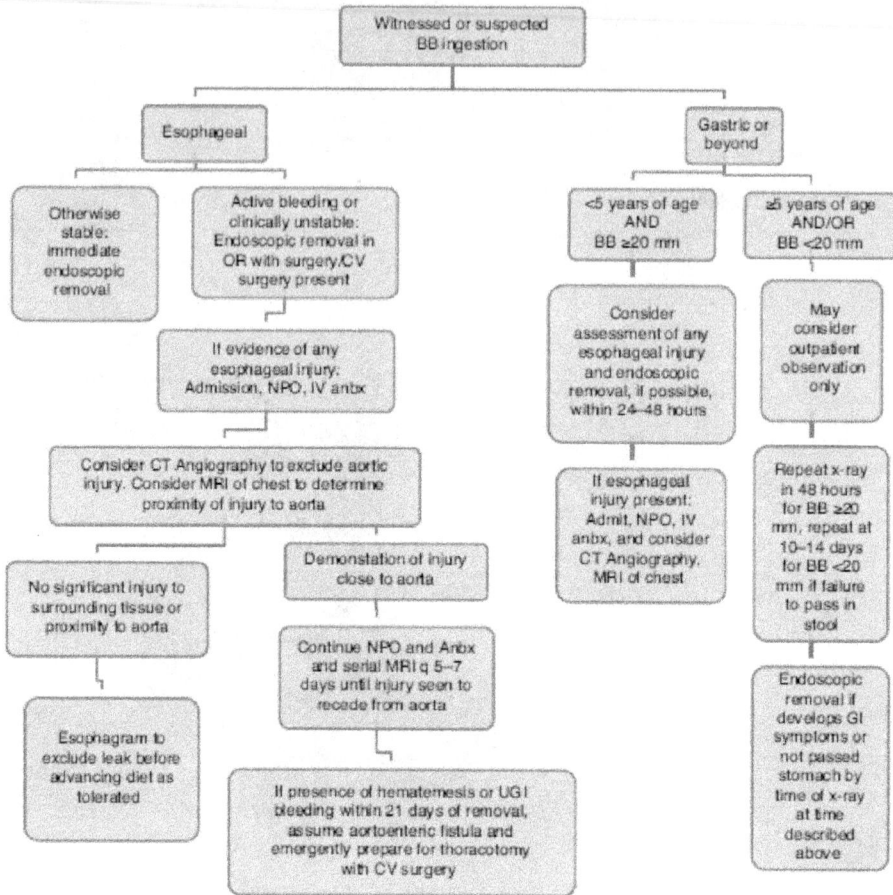

Figure 2.
Kramer's algorithm of BB ingestion.

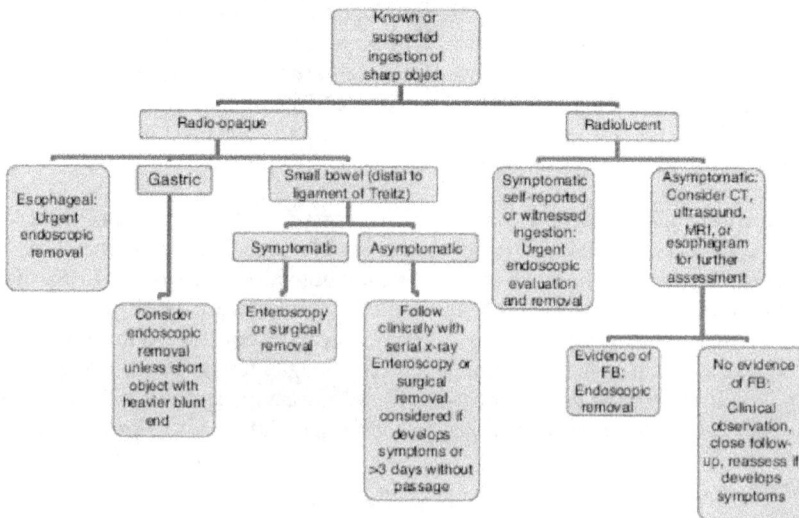

Figure 3.
Kramer's algorithm of sharp object ingestion.

Initial presentation

-Obtain history
  -Known magnet ingestion
  -Unexplained GI symptoms with rare earth magnets in environment
-Obtain an abdominal x-ray. If magnets are present on flat plate, obtain lateral x-ray
-Determine single versus multiple magnet ingestion

Single magnet

Multiple magnet (or single magnet and metallic object)

Within the stomach or esophagus
-Option 1: Consult Pediatric GI if available.
-Consider removal if patient at increased risk for further ingestion
-Option 2: Follow serial x-rays as outpatient and educate parents*

Beyond the stomach
-Consult pediatric GI if available.
-Consider removal if possible.
-Follow with serial x-rays as outpatient
-Educate parents*
-Confirm passage with serial x-ray
-If delayed progression, may use PEG 3350 or other laxative to aid passage

All within the stomach or esophagus
-If pediatric GI available, notify for removal, especially if <12 hours
-If not available, transfer to referral center
-If >12 hours until time of procedure, then consult pediatric surgery prior to endoscopic removal

Beyond the stomach
-Consult pediatric GI and pediatric surgeon if available
-If not available, send to referral center
-Management depends on whether symptomatic or asymptomatic

Successful removal
-Discharge home with follow-up and education

Unsuccessful removal
-Refer to surgery for removal

Symptomatic
-Refer to pediatric surgery

Asymptomatic
-If no obstruction or perforation on x-ray, may remove by enteroscopy or colonoscopy if available or follow with serial x-ray
-May do serial x-ray in ED to check for progression every 4–6 hours

Successful endoscopic removal
-Discharge after feeding tolerance, with appropriate follow-up and education

***Parental education:**
-Remove any magnetic objects nearby
-Avoid clothes with metallic buttons or belts with buckles
-Ensure no other metal objects or magnets are in the child environment for accidental ingestion

No progression on serial x-rays
-Admit for further monitoring and serial x-rays or surgical removal
-May use PEG 3350 or other laxative to aid in passage and to help prepare for colonoscopy
-Continue serial x-ray every 8–12 hours. If no symptoms, then proceed with surgical removal or endoscopic removal with surgical backup

Progression of magnets on serial x-rays
-Educate parents on precautions* and discharge with close follow-up
-Confirm passage with serial x-rays
-If at any time magnets do not progress or patient becomes symptomatic, admit to hospital for removal of magnets

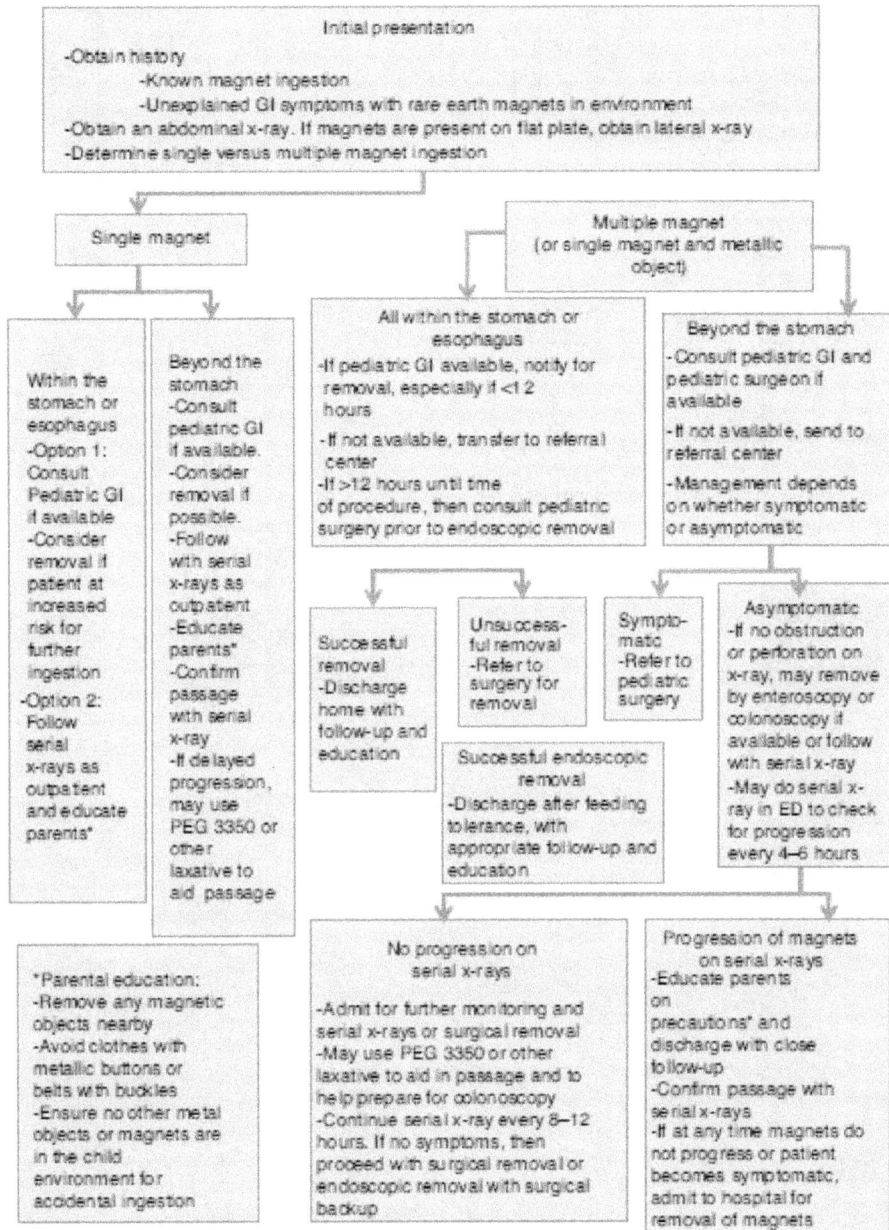

Figure 4.
Kramer's algorithm of magnet ingestion.

or magnet with a metallic FB are located within the esophagus or the stomach, these FBs must be endoscopically removed [27]. Symptomatic children with either multiple magnets or a single magnet with a metallic FB in any site of the digestive system need to consult a pediatric surgeon (**Figure 4**) [22].

6.5 Bezoars

Management of Phytobezoar may resolve spontaneously over weeks to months. Small feedings containing digestive or mucolytic enzymes (several types of chemical dissolution or prokinetic agents as cotazym, viokase, or mucomyst) may use if there is no outlet obstruction. If the bezoar is symptomatic in large objects or does not dissolve, extraction by endoscopic or surgical removal is recommended. In medication Bezoars, Gastric lavage with saline is usually effective is dissolving the bezoar within ten days [24, 25].

7. Conclusion

Although some cases of ingestion of FBs are dangerous and require surgical intervention, educating parents about the risk of swallowing FBs remains the most important procedure in the prevention.

Acknowledgements

We wish to thank the medical officer, and the doctors in the Pediatrics. department.

Conflict of interest

None declared.

Author details

Leen Jamel Doya[1*] and Ali Ibrahim[2]

1 Department of Pediatrics, Tishreen University Hospital, Latakia, Syria

2 Department of Pediatrics, Professor of Gastroenterology and Hepatology, Tishreen University Hospital, Lattakia, Syria

*Address all correspondence to: dr.leen.doya@gmail.com

IntechOpen

References

[1] Lee, M., and S. C. Kim. Appendiceal foreign body in an infant. Medicine 2017;96(17): e6717. DOI: http://dx.doi.org/10.1097/MD.0000000000006717

[2] Lee JH. Foreign body ingestion in children. Clinical endoscopy 2018;51(2):129-136. DOI: http://dx.doi.org/ 10.5946/ce.2018.039.

[3] Seo, J. K. Endoscopic management of gastrointestinal foreign bodies in children. Indian journal of pediatrics. 1999; 66(1):S75-80. PMID: 11132474

[4] Orsagh-Yentis D, McAdams RJ, Roberts KJ, LB MK. Foreign-body ingestions of young children treated in US emergency departments: 1995-2015. Pediatrics. 2019;143(5):e20181988. DOI: https://doi.org/10.1542/peds.2018-1988

[5] Hesham AKH. Foreign body ingestion: children like to put objects in their mouth. World J Pediatr. 2010;6(4):301-310. Doi:10.1007/s12519-010-0231-y

[6] Jayachandra S, Eslick GD. A systematic review of paediatric foreign body ingestion: presentation, complications, and management. Int J Pediatr Otorhinolaryngol. 2013;77(3):311-317. Doi:10.1016/j.ijporl.2012.11.025

[7] Ikenberry S.O, Jue T.L, Anderson M.A, Appalaneni V, Banerjee S, Ben-Menachem T, et al.Management of ingested foreign bodies and food impactions. Gastrointestinal endoscopy. 2011; 73(6):1085-1091. DOI: 10.1016/j.gie.2010.11.010

[8] Gregori D, Scarinzi C, Morra B, Salerni L, Berchialla P, Snidero S, et al. Ingested foreign bodies causing complications and requiring hospitalization in European children: Results from the ESFBI study. Pediatr Int. 2010;52(1):26-32. Doi:10.1111/j.1442-200X.2009.02862.x

[9] Lee BK, Ryu HH, Moon JM, Jeung KW. Bowel perforations induced by multiple magnet ingestion. Emerg Med Australas 2010;22(2):189-191. Doi:10.1111/j.1742-6723.2010.01276.x

[10] Sola Jr R, Rosenfeld E.H, Yangyang R.Y, Peter S.D.S, Shah S.R. Magnet foreign body ingestion: rare occurrence but big consequences. Journal of pediatric surgery. 2018; 53(9):1815-1819. Doi:10.1016/j.jpedsurg.2017.08.013.

[11] Khorana J, Tantivit Y, Phiuphong C, Pattapong S, Siripan S. Foreign body ingestion in pediatrics: distribution, management and complications. Medicina. 2019; 55(10):686-690. doi:10.3390/medicina55100686

[12] Gurevich Y, Sahn B, Weinstein T. Foreign body ingestion in pediatric patients. Current opinion in pediatrics. 2018; 30(5): 677-682. doi: 10.5946/ce.2018.039

[13] Waltzman M.L, Baskin M, Wypij D, Mooney D, Jones D, Fleisher G. A randomized clinical trial of the management of esophageal coins in children. Pediatrics. 2005; 116(3): 614-619. Doi:10.1542/peds.2004-2555

[14] Singh N, Chong J, Ho J, Jayachandra S, Cope D, Azimi F, Wong E. Predictive factors associated with spontaneous passage of coins: A ten-year analysis of paediatric coin ingestion in Australia. International journal of pediatric otorhinolaryngology. 2018; 113(1): 266-271. doi:10.1016/j.ijporl.2018.08.010

[15] Litovitz T, Whitaker N, Clark L, White N.C, Marsolek M. Emerging battery-ingestion hazard: clinical implications. Pediatrics. 2010; 125(6): 1168-1177. DOI: 10.1542/peds.2009-3037

[16] Krom H, Visser M, Hulst J.M, Wolters V.M, Van den Neucker A.M,

de Meij T Kindermann A. Serious complications after button battery ingestion in children. European journal of pediatrics. 2018;177(7): 1063-1070. Doi:10.1007/s00431-018-3154-6

[17] Eliason M.J, Ricca R.L, Gallagher T.Q. Button battery ingestion in children. Current opinion in otolaryngology & head and neck surgery. 2017; 25(6): 520-526. Doi:10.1097/MOO.0000000 000000410

[18] Jatana K.R, Litovitz T, Reilly J.S, Koltai P.J, Rider G, Jacobs I.N. Pediatric button battery injuries: 2013 task force update. International journal of pediatric otorhinolaryngology. 2013; 77(9):1392-1399. Doi:10.1016/j.ijporl.2013.06.006

[19] Alzahem A.M, Soundappan S.S, Jefferies H, Cass D.T. Ingested magnets and gastrointestinal complications. Journal of paediatrics and child health. 2007; 43(6): 497-498. Doi:10.1111/j.1440-1754.2007.01121.x

[20] Diaz R, Davalos G, Welsh L.K, Portenier D, Guerron A.D. Use of magnets in gastrointestinal surgery. Surgical endoscopy. 2019; 33(6): 1721-1730. doi:10.1007/s00464-019-06718-w

[21] Palta R, Sahota A, Bemarki A, Salama P, Simpson N, Laine L. Foreign-body ingestion: characteristics and outcomes in a lower socioeconomic population with predominantly intentional ingestion. Gastrointestinal endoscopy. 2009; 69(3):426-433. doi:10.1016/j.gie.2008.05.072

[22] Lee J.H, Lee J.S, Kim M.J, Choe Y.H. Initial location determines spontaneous passage of foreign bodies from the gastrointestinal tract in children. Pediatric emergency care. 2011; 27(4): 284-289. doi: 10.1097/PEC.0b013e 318213131a

[23] Campos R.R, Paricio P.P, Albasini J.A, Riquelme J.R, Tebar J.C, Mompeán, J.L, Ayllón J.G. Gastrointestinal Bezoars. Digestive surgery. 1990; 7(1): 39-44. doi:10.1159/000171939.

[24] AlMuhsin A.M., Alsalman F, Bubshait A, Hajar R.O.A. Surgical Management of Massive Metal Bezoar. Cureus. 2021; 13(1): 1-5. doi: 10.7759/cureus.12597

[25] Andrus C.H, Ponsky J.L. Bezoars: classification, pathophysiology, and treatment. American Journal of Gastroenterology. 1988;83(5):476-478. PMID: 3284334

[26] Leinwand K, Brumbaugh D.E, Kramer R.E. Button Battery Ingestion in Children: A Paradigm for Management of Severe Pediatric Foreign Body Ingestions. Gastrointestinal endoscopy clinics of North America. 2016; 26(1): 99-118. Doi:10.1016/j.giec.2015.08.003

[27] Hussain S.Z, Bousvaros A, Gilger M, Mamula P, Gupta S, Kramer R, Noel R.A. Management of ingested magnets in children. Journal of pediatric gastroenterology and nutrition. 2012; 55(3): 239-242. doi: 10.1097/MPG.0b013e3182687be0

Chapter 4

Bowel Anastomoses: Manual or Mechanical

Alpha Oumar Toure, Mamadou Seck,
Mohamadou Lamine Gueye and Ousmane Thiam

Abstract

An anastomosis is a connection between two tubular anatomical structures. Anastomoses have been a great surgical challenge from antiquities to modern times. Main research on the manual techniques and healing processes of digestive anastomoses took place during the 19th century. They were later improved by the advent of mechanical devices in the early 20th century. For both types of anastomoses, local and general conditions required for a good healing are the same. Many devices, both for manual and mechanical anastomoses have been developed. The devices' uses depend on their availability, surgeons usual practice and the relative difficulty of the anastomosis. The debate is still lively about the advantages and the potential inconveniences of one technique versus the other in regards to many parameters such as operating time and the incidence of anastomotic leakage.

Keywords: bowel, anastomosis, manual, stapled, outcomes

1. Introduction

Many methods of intestinal anastomoses have been performed since the earliest days of surgery, from the manual anastomoses that were developed in the 19th century to our days where stapled anastomoses are gaining significant popularity. The results of studies comparing the two techniques are still contradictory and cannot prove one's superiority over the other. Our objective in this chapter is to present a brief review of the history of bowel anastomosis, bowel healing process, and comprehensive comparison of hand-sewn and mechanical bowel anastomoses.

2. Historical aspects

Anastomosis is a connection between two solid or hollow structures. Performing a digestive anastomosis has long represented a major challenge in surgical practice, and as early as the 19th century, it was established that the first-line digestive healing required edge-to-edge facing of the walls in a sealed and hemostatic manner. The work of Antoine Lembert in 1826 had established "as a dogma" the need to oppose the serosa by inverting the digestive tunics using needles set with silk thread or catgut [1]. This theory was then questioned few months later by the Belgian Henroz, who proved the feasibility of an anastomosis by eversion using rings [1]. Europe was thus the region of abundant research on digestive anastomoses. In 1887,

Halsted demonstrated the importance of the submucosal layer as the only solid structure that guarantees the watertightness of the assembly [2]. While a large trend was for sutures to be fashioned in two planes (mucosa by overlock and sero-muscular at separate points), it is to the brave tenacity of Pierre Jourdan that we owe the possibility of performing the bowel anastomosis in one plane which according to the author "held on very well" [3]. Few years later across the Atlantic, Orr clearly showed in 1969 that continuous overlock suturing in one plane was effective and safe. This message was then confirmed by several other authors [4–6]. Experimental work on the manual techniques continued to develop until the 1980s, focusing both on the type of material to use and on how to deal with the digestive tunics.

Along with the development of manual suturing, mechanical technique was also the subject of much work. In 1892, John Murphy of Chicago developed a two-button cholecysto-jejunal anastomosis technique, which was later extended to other digestive structures [7]. Most of the principles of mechanical stapling were laid down by the Hungarian Hult in 1909: compression of the tissues, form of B-staples, staggered arrangement of staples [8]. Von Petz developed in 1921 a device widely used for gastric stapling, later improved by the Japanese Nakayama [9, 10]. The former USSR contributed to the development of the mechanical stapling devices by the end of World War II. In a very large and war-torn country, it was necessary to develop easy to teach techniques for poorly trained surgeons. The research institute then created linear and circular staplers, efficient but too heavy in steel [11]. In 1958, returning from a study trip to Ukraine, American Mark Ravitch developed the technique in his laboratory in Baltimore, first on the lungs, then extended to other surgeries. He founded a company in order to establish, with his students, an entire successful range of mechanical anastomosis equipment whose main advances were: lighter and more manageable instruments, staggered staples already pre-installed and sterilized allowing several uses with the same forceps. In 1976, the first single-use mechanical stapler was marketed. Numerous technical developments contributed to the progressive improvement in the devices such as articulated grippers, and replacement of the stainless steel of the clips with a biocompatible titanium alloy [12].

3. Anastomosis healing BASIS

The healing of a digestive anastomosis is achieved through tissue regeneration processes that respond to the general laws of inflammation [13]. It does not therefore depend directly on the suturing technique. The digestive gap created will be filled in three successive stages:

1. A loose edematous infiltrate, following the vascular response to trauma: after immediate formation of a platelet nail, secondary vasodilation allows the influx of pro-inflammatory substances (histamine and prostaglandins) and the release of proteolytic substances; A cellular influx occurs in the following hours in the form of polynuclear neutrophils, macrophages then fibroblasts, cells resulting from the interstitial tissue and differentiated locally in order to produce fibrin, key element of the solidity.

2. A cellular granulation tissue then appears towards cicatricial sclerosis allowing restoration ad integrum or with a local scar.

3. Re-epithelialization begins very early (approximately 24 hours) after trauma. The mucous layer and basement membrane thicken at the wound and the

basal cells migrate to the wound, dividing and producing daughter cells. The reconstituted mucous layer is thus thinner at the level of the scar and rests on a fibrinous support frame.

The healing process is then influenced by many factors of two categories; local and general [14]:

- Local factors:

  o *The Parietal breach* is the most dependent on surgical technique. Too much stitch spacing or improper contact creates spaces that are difficult for the granulation tissue to fill.

  o *Alteration of the granulation tissue* depends on many factors such as the extent of the necrosis, the inclusion of foci of mucous membrane and intestinal germs, the foreign body reaction to the sutures or staples.

  o *Infection* modifies the healing phenomena through enzymatic reactions altering the quality of local collagen.

- General factors

Several other factors are often neglected; however, they contribute to the quality of healing. These include the nutritional status, the defensive capacity and hemodynamic status of the patient. A digestive anastomosis should be omitted in the events of hemodynamic failure, significant patient undernutrition, significant inflammation, generalized sepsis, advanced cancer, and emergency interventions for generalized peritonitis, intestinal obstruction, or significant fecal contamination. Likewise, the presence of patient-specific immunosuppressive factors such as chronic smoking, diabetes or long-term corticosteroid therapy may prompt surgeons to either giving up performing an anastomosis, or postponing it, and/or protecting it with a temporary diverting enterostomy. These risk factors are potentially responsible for real changes in the operating strategy and must be communicated to the patient before the procedure.

- Surgical technical factors:

  o The ABSENCE OF ANY TENSION is easily achieved for mobile structures like the small intestine

  o The ANASTOMOTIC EDGES MUST BE WELL VASCULARIZED, both arterially and venously.

  o VALID ENTEROSYNTHESIS PROCESS (MANUAL OR MECHANICAL): the manual anastomosis technique must be of high quality and it is only at this precise point that the surgeon influences the quality of healing. Mechanical stapling pliers must be reliable. Two checks are useful after anastomosis: the quality control of the flanges in case of circular stapling, the airtightness test which seems useful but not essential [15];

  o HEMOSTASE OF ANASTOMOTIC SEGMENTS: Local bleeding can activate proteolytic enzymes and damage local granulation tissue. However, this last point could be in contradiction with the good vascularization of the tissues:

it is therefore necessary to find the right compromise and not to excessively electro-coagulate the digestive walls. Hemostasis with fine threads or bipolar forceps is often very useful for this purpose [15].

4. Types of anastomoses

Digestive anastomoses are designated after the two types of viscera involved (esophagus, stomach, jejunum, ileum, colon, rectum, bile duct), and, on the way in which the stoma mouths are anastomosed. The term "terminal" (T) is used when the entire mouth of the bowel is involved with the anastomosis, and the term "lateral" (L) when the side of the bowel segment and not its mouths is incorporated into the anastomosis. There are thus four types of anastomosis:

- End-to-end (TT) when the two digestive segments are "mouth-to-mouth" anastomosis.

- Terminolateral (TL) when the mouth of the first designated segment is anasto-mosed on the side of the second designated segment.

- Lateroterminal (LT): the reverse of the previous one.

- Laterolateral (LL) when the two segments are anastomosed side by side, the ends requiring elective closure. This is referred to as a "terminal" LL anastomosis.

Thus, a "terminal colorectal" anastomosis is the opening of the colonic mouth on the anterior or posterior surface of the rectum, while a "lateroterminal colorectal" anastomosis is the connection from the lateral surface of the colon to the rectal mouth.

- Hand-sewn anastomoses

Traditionally, anastomoses were hand-sewn. The two-layer technique generated a certain sense of security in the past but single-layer anastomoses are now pre-ferred because they heal faster. In fact, they allow a more accurate musculo-mucosal realignment and cause less reduction in lumen size and less tissue strangulation than two-layer techniques [16].
Interrupted single-layer serosubmucosal suture is the preferred hand-sewn tech-nique. Interrupted sero-submucosal sutures allow the best tissue apposition and cause minimal damage to the submucosal vascularization.
Continuous single-layer serosubmucosal suture is particularly effective if digestive tract's access is good and the anastomosis is technically simple as in the upper gastro-intestinal tract (gastro- jejunostomy and bilio-enteric anastomoses). It is preferred to the interrupted single-layer technique in these cases because it is quicker [16].
Monofilament threads (like polydioxanone) are preferred because they usually cause less fibrosis formation than the braided ones (polyglactin). It has been noted that more inflammation is likely to happen in the braided suture lines. Local edema can lead to increased digestive transit difficulty and colicky pain [17].

- Stapled anastomoses

Three types of suturing devices have been developed: non-cutting linear suturing forceps, cutting linear suturing forceps and circular suturing forceps. However, there exists a great diversity of materials currently available in the market that are being constant upgraded. Staplers are appealing because they are easy to use and may be quicker than some sutured anastomoses. In situations where anastomosis is difficult (low colorectal) or if multiple anastomoses are required at the end of a lengthy procedure, mechanical devices can be very useful. The anatomy of the stapled intestinal anastomosis is similar to traditional two-layer hand-sewn anastomosis and they require the same attention as hand-sewn anastomoses. Anastomoses can be made with linear or circular stapling devices, used alone or in combination. The choice of a technique (triangulation with a cutting or non-cutting linear forceps, combined use of cutting and non-cutting forceps, use of a circular forceps) is made by the surgeon during the operation. This choice depends on the dimensions of the tissue, in particular their thickness, the diameter of the viscera to be anastomosed and their site (deep or superficial anastomosis in abdominal surgery). The use of mechanical sutures respects the main principles of classical surgery, with its indications, precautions for use and contraindications [18].

- Sutureless anastomoses

They have been in use since Murphy's button in 1892 [19]. Nowadays, sutureless devices include compression magnetic rings, tissue glue, laser-YAG or self-gripping mesh. But most of these techniques remain experimental [20–22].

5. Choice between manual and mechanical anastomoses

The choice of anastomotic technique is between hand-sewn sutures and staples, because sutureless anastomoses remain experimental. The selection of technique is often made on the grounds of personal convenience, cost, and personal experience. Objective evidence has failed to show an outstanding benefit that would favor the use of staples over manual sutures. Most randomized trials comparing a variety of suture techniques with staples did not confirm the advantage of stapled anastomoses in terms of leaks, mortality or cancer recurrence. The increased rate of stapled anastomoses stenosis is well documented. Only few strictures require treatment, usually by dilation or endoluminal incision/resection. Surgeons in training should adopt an anastomotic method that is easily reproducible. Hand-sewn single-layer techniques (continuous or interrupted) should be mastered before relying on stapling devices, allowing the surgeon to take action if technical problems occur with stapling.

Stapled intestinal anastomoses have been widely studied and are preferred over hand-sewn anastomoses because of their safety and efficacy profiles [23–25]. There is evidence suggesting that decreased operative time and anastomotic leak rates may be associated with the use of a stapled technique, in some types of anastomoses such as ileocolic anastomosis [26]. Overall, the evidence that is available has shown no difference between stapled and hand-sewn anastomotic techniques [27–30]. Stapled anastomoses are supposed to take less time, therefore, the operative stress on the patient should be lower leading to faster recovery with lower rate of postoperative ileus and shorter hospital stay as Bragg et al. could show in their study (operating time $p = 0,02$; anastomotic failures $p = 0,03$; hospital days $p < 0,01$) [31]. Jurowich et al., compared stapled versus hand-sewn anastomoses in 4062 patients with right sided hemicolectomy due to right colon cancer, published similar results even though less operating time did not translate into shorter overall hospital stay in that study [31]. The occurrence of post-operative ileus also depends on the extent of the resection, the intraoperative fluid management, the use of minimally-invasive surgery versus open surgery and many more factors. It is the combination of many of those parameters that contribute to the development of postoperative ileus and therefore a consecutive prolonged hospital stay [31–33].

Higher hospital readmission rate after bowel resection is often associated with anastomotic leakage [34]. Some authors showed a 30-day readmission rate around 10% after hand-sewn colo-rectal surgery, slightly higher than those with stapled anastomoses [35]. Determining the type of anastomosis (stapled or hand-sewn) which may lead to a reduced risk of anastomotic leak is still a matter of debate. On one hand, some authors like Farrah et al., showed a 2-times elevated risk of developing anastomotic leakage after stapled anastomoses compared to hand-sewn anastomoses. Nordholm-Carstens et al. in Denmark, conducted a retrospective cohort study that found 5.4% anastomotic leaks in the stapled versus 2.4% leaks in the hand-sewn group, this was statistically significant ($p = 0.004$) [36]. In contrast, Choy et al., in a Cochrane Database Review, showed a significantly lower anastomotic leakage rate in stapled anastomoses. These conflicting results may be attributed to the different ways of performing the stapled and sutured anastomosis, varying stapling and suture material and varying experience of the surgical team [37–39].

Performing perfect anastomoses is, of course, associated with higher levels of training and experience of the surgeon. It has always been a subject of discussion if and which anastomoses can be safely performed by an intern or surgical trainee. Schineis et al. in Germany provided some evidence that bowel anastomosis can be as safely performed by a surgical trainee as by a more experienced surgeon [40]. Cost is one of the major concerns that may prohibit the use of stapling devices. The impact of the use of stapling devices on hospitals' costs has rarely been explored. Devices cost may differ from hospital to another due to individual contracts negotiated between the individual hospitals and the distributing industries, it also varies between different countries [40].

6. Conclusion

There is a lot of debate around the choice of hand-sewn versus stapled intestinal anastomosis in view of multiple variables such as surgeon's convenience and experience, results concerning hospital length of stay and occurrence of anastomotic leakage. Stapled anastomoses seem to be favored compared to hand-sewn anastomoses in terms of operation time, cost in the operating rooms and total hospital costs in many studies on adult patients. Finally, it is up to the surgeons, in accordance to their usual practice and their individual patients' needs, to choose one technique over the other.

Author details

Alpha Oumar Toure*, Mamadou Seck, Mohamadou Lamine Gueye
and Ousmane Thiam
Surgery and Surgical Specialties Department, Cheikh Anta Diop University,
Dakar, Senegal

*Address all correspondence to: alpha.oumar@yahoo.fr

IntechOpen

References

[1] Lembert A. Mémoire sur l'enterroraphie. Rep Gen Anat Physiol Pathol 1826; 2:101.

[2] Halsted XS. Circular suture of the intestine. An experimental study. J 1887;103:245-7.

[3] Jourdan P. Sutures en un plan des tuniques digestives. Position actuelle. J Chir 1965;90:649-55.

[4] Orr NW. A single-layer intestinal anastomosis. Br J Surg 1969;56:771-4.

[5] Gambee LP, Garnjobst W, Hardwick CE. Ten years' experience of a single-layer anastomosis in colonic surgery. Am J Surg 1956;92:222-7.

[6] Everett WG. A comparison of one layer and two layer techniques for colorectal anastomosis. Br J Surg 1975;62:135-40.

[7] Murphy JB. Intestinal approximation, with special reference to the use of the anastomosis button. Lancet 1894;2:621.

[8] Hultl 2nd H. Kongress der Ungarischen Gesellschaft für Chirurgie. Budapest. Mai 1908. Pester Med Chir 1909;45:108 [10,121-2]

[9] Von Petz A. Aseptic technique of stomach resections. Ann Surg 1927;86:338-43.

[10] Nakayama K. Simplification of the Bilroth I gastric resection. Surgery 1954;35:837-41.

[11] Androssov PI. Experience in the application of the instrumental mechanical suture in surgery of the stomach and rectum. Acta Chir Scand 1970;136:57-63.

[12] F.M. Steichen. Naissance des sutures mécaniques modernes en chirurgie: petites et grandes histoires, en hommage à Mark Ravitch. Chirurgie 1998, 123(6): 616-623.

[13] Wind GG, Rich NM. Principles of surgical technique. The art of surgery. Munchen: Urban and Scharzenberg; 1987.

[14] Welter R, Patel JC. Chirurgie mécanique digestive. Paris: Masson; 1985.

[15] Kwon S, Morris A, Billingham R, Frankhouse J, Horvath K, Johnson M, et al., for the Surgical Care an Outcomes Assessment Program (SCOAP) Collaborative. Routine leak testing in colorectal surgery in the surgical care and outcomes assessment program. Arch Surg 2012;147:345-51.

[16] McKinley AJ, Krukowski ZH. Intestinal amastomoses. Surgery 2006, 24(7): 224-8.

[17] Marques dos Santos CH et al. Differences between polydioxanone and polyglactin in intestinal anastomoses – a comparative study of intestinal anastomoses. J Coloproctol 2017, 37(4):263-267.

[18] Nuiry O, Pedroli E, Simoens X, Balique JG. Les sutures mécaniques. Pharm. Hosp 1990;(101):7-15.

[19] M'ardle, J.S. The position of Murphy's button in modern surgery. Trans RAM Ireland 1900, 18:145.

[20] Jamshidi R, Stephenson JT, Clay JG, Pichakron KO, Harrison MR. Magnamosis: magnetic compression anastomosis with comparison to suture and staple techniques. Journal of Pediatric Surgery 2009, 44(1): 222-228.

[21] Yao L, Li C, Zhu X, Shao Y, Meng S, Shi L, Wang H. An Effective New

Intestinal Anastomosis Method. Med Sci Monit. 2016;22:4570-4576.

[22] Chao Fan et al. Sutureless Intestinal Anastomosis with a Novel Device of Magnetic Compression Anastomosis. Chinese Medical Sciences Journal 2011, 26(3): 182-189.

[23] Goulder F. Bowel anastomoses: The theory, the practice and the evidence base. World J Gastrointest Surg 2012;4:208-13.

[24] Neutzling CB, Lustosa SA, Da Silva EM, et al. Stapled versus handsewn methods for colorectal anastomosis surgery. Cochrane Database Syst Rev 2012;15:CD003144.

[25] Slieker JC, Daams F, Mulder IM, et al. Systematic Review of the Technique of Colorectal Anastomosis. JAMA Surg 2013;148:190-201.

[26] Choy PY, Bissett IP, Docherty JG, et al. Stapled versus handsewn methods for ileocolic anastomoses. Cochrane Database Syst Rev 2011;7:CD004320.

[27] Wrighton L, Curtis JL, Gollin G. Stapled intestinal anastomoses in infants. J Pediatr Surg 2008;43:2231-4.

[28] Mitchell IC, Barber R, Fischer AC, et al. Experience performing 64 consecutive stapled intestinal anastomoses in small children and infants. J Pediatr Surg 2011;46:128-30.

[29] Powell RW. Stapled intestinal anastomosis in neonates and infants: use of the endoscopic intestinal stapler. J Pediatr Surg 1995;30:195-7.

[30] Simmons JD, Gunter III JW, Manley JD, et al. Stapled intestinal anastomosis in neo- nates. Am Surg 2010;76:644-6.

[31] Jurowich C, Lichthardt S, Matthes N, Kastner C, Haubitz I, Prock A, et al. Effects of anastomotic technique on early postoperative outcome in open right-sided hemicolectomy. BJS Open 2019;3:203e7.

[32] Bragg D, El-Sharkawy AM, Psaltis E, Maxwell-Armstrong CA, Lobo DN. Postoperative ileus: recent developments in pathophysiology and management. Clin Nutr 2015;34:367e76.

[33] Farrah JP, Lauer CW, Bray MS, McCartt JM, Chang MC, Meredith JW, Miller PR, Mowery NT. Stapled versus hand-sewn anastomoses in emergency general surgery: a retrospective review of outcomes in a unique patient population. J Trauma Acute Care Surg. 2013;74(5):1187-92.

[34] Midura E, Hanseman D, Davis B, Atkinson S, Abbott D, Shah S, et al. Risk factors and consequences of anastomotic leak after colectomy: a national analysis. Dis *Colon rectum* 2015;58:333e8.

[35] Al-Mazrou AM, Suradkar K, Mauro CM, Kiran RP. Characterization of readmission by day of rehospitalization after colorectal surgery. Dis *Colon rectum* 2017;60:202e12.

[36] Nordholm-Carstensen A, Schnack Rasmussen M, Krarup P-M. Increased leak rates following stapled versus handsewn ileocolic anastomosis in patients with right-sided colon cancer: a nationwide cohort study. Dis *Colon rectum* 2019;62:542e50.

[37] Resegotti A, Astegiano M, Farina E, Ciccone G, Avagnina G, Giustetto A, et al. "Side-to-side stapled anastomosis strongly reduces anastomotic leak rates in Crohn's disease surgery". Dis *Colon rectum* Mar. 2005;48:464e8.

[38] Morse B et al. Determination of independent predictive factors for anastomotic leak: analysis of 682 intestinal anastomoses The American Journal of Surgery 2013; 206:950-956.

[39] Hintz GC, Alshehri A, Bell CM, Butterworth SA. Stapled versus hand-sewn pediatric intestinal anastomoses: a retrospective cohort study. Journal of Pediatric Surgery 2018, 53:959-963.

[40] Schineis et al. stapled intestinal anastomoses are more cost effective than hand-sewn anastomoses in a diagnosis related group system. The Surgeon 2020, https://doi.org/10.1016/j.surge.2020.09.002

Chapter 5

Postoperative Follow-Up and Recovery after Abdominal Surgery

Stelian Stefanita Mogoanta, Stefan Paitici
and Carmen Aurelia Mogoanta

Abstract

Postoperative patient care has several components: - surveillance, – prevention of complications associated with surgical disease or other preexisting comorbidities, – specific postoperative treatment of the surgical disease and its complications. While these distinctions are purely didactic, the postoperative care merges into an active surveillance with a higher level of standardization than it would seem at first glance. Computing, interpreting and integrating signs and symptoms with active search of proofs by lab tests or other paraclinical explorations highly depends on skills and dedication of the entire healthcare team. Those attributes gained through continuous theoretical preparation but validated by current practice bring added value, always in favor of the patients' best interests. In this chapter, we propose to explore the main clinical and paraclinical means and tools that can improve the outcomes of surgical procedures for a faster and safer recovery. We will also discuss the need for different types of surgical bed drains placement and their management, the use of antibiotics and thrombotic event prophylaxis.

Keywords: postoperative, follow-up, surgery, complication, prophylaxis, treatment

1. Introduction

The surgical act, defined as the time that a surgeon effectively operates on the patient, remains the center of surgical therapy, however, it is increasingly clear that the preoperative and more importantly the postoperative care can enhance or unfortunately compromise the results of a technically successful surgery. For reducing the mortality and morbidity rates in the postoperative period, it is crucial to identify risk factors, prevent and treat as soon as possible any deviation of the patient state from the normal rehabilitation course. Timely interventions reduce the impact of the negative events in the patient's recovery. Early recognition of signs and symptoms by close surveillance is the key and starting point for active surveillance. This allows targeted lab testing or imaging (if needed) to rapidly identify any undesired event in patient recovery and allow for specific and proper action.

2. Fever

To monitor the operated patient, we have at our disposal the clinical and paraclinical parameters. The patient's **temperature,** despite being a general and non-specific parameter, is one of the most important and easy to monitor.

During the follow-up period of the surgical patient, the temperature is usually measured at least twice a day, in the morning and in the afternoon, and whenever there is a suspicion of fever. The determinations are included in the observation sheet completing the temperature graph whose oscillations become suggestive in a clinical context. A single febrile rise, below 38 degrees Celsius can often be caused by the resorption of blood degradation products from the operative wound or secondary to the excessive maintenance of a drainage tube, without major pathological significance [1]. However, the persistence of the fever with the configuration of "saw teeth" on the thermal chart suggests the development of a septic process. The first to be checked is the surgical site, then the lung and urinary system, as these are the most frequent sites of infection after surgery. Particular attention should be paid to the occult causes of fever such as endocarditis, phlebitis, lamellar atelectasis that should be systematically searched for in the context of an unjustified febrile syndrome with an apparently good evolution in the operative site. In a large cohort study [2], the most common causes of fever development were stratified a few days after surgery. On the day of surgery, cardiac pathology and specific myocardial infarction seem to be the most common, then pulmonary pathology – pneumonia and atelectasis seem to cause fever in days 1–3 postoperatively. Urinary infections usually occur in 2–3 days postoperatively but can also begin later. From day 4 to 30 postoperatively, superficial or profound surgical site infections become the main cause for fever development, while thrombosis can cause fever at any time between the day of surgery and postoperative day 30. When the febrile ascension appears suddenly on the fifth day after surgery, without signs of wound infection anastomosis dehiscence should be suspected, however, it can also be caused by thrombophlebitis. Therefore, we can conclude that fever is a general sign that should always be interpreted in accordance with other signs and symptoms but it is an alarming sign that should lead to careful and complete physical examination and laboratory tests or imaging studies evaluated on a case-by-case basis.

3. Supervision of the cardiovascular system

Cardiovascular system stability is crucial in the postoperative evolution of the patient. Complex surveillance is needed in many cases and the rehabilitation measures must be intensive and prompt, conducted in most cases by the intensive care specialist or cardiologist. However, the surgeon must be prepared to recognize cardiac risks and main syndromes and even manage the patient until one of the above mentioned specialists are available.

Heart rate is systematically monitored several times a day. Immediately postoperatively, the pulse rate is usually higher than normal with a decreased amplitude, may be justified by intra operative blood loss, which may remain insignificant in the overall economy of the patient's healing, or by anesthetic drugs, the extent of surgical "aggressiveness", pain, etc. As these factors are progressively corrected, the heart rate should return to normal. Additional oxygen administration can help achieve a faster normal rate as it improves tissue oxygenation [3]. It is very important to compare the pulse frequency with the values noted preoperatively taking into account the patient's underlying pathology (thyroid, heart, etc.). The pulse with increasing frequency from one determination to another, with a small amplitude that becomes progressively filiform, associated with hypotension in a sweaty and pale patient, may be caused by a bleeding at the operating site (which is not always in the drain tube or in the container); this may require analysis of reoperation for hemostatic purposes. Tachycardia with low pulse amplitude and a decrease in blood pressure that occurs on days 4–6 postoperatively, may indicate a septic complication or anastomosis dehiscence. On the other hand, bradycardia is however associated with increased cardiac, pulmonary, renal and pain-related morbidity at 3 and 5 days after surgery [4]. The discovery of arrhythmias whether extrasystolic or atrial fibrillation as a new event, requires rapid correction of ionic and hydric imbalances and the search for a septic process, the most likely causes in this context. Both bradycardia and arrythmias always require a postoperative cardiac consult [4, 5].

Blood pressure is determined at least twice a day. The recorded values are interpreted in a dynamic clinical context, always compared with the normal values of the patient determined preoperatively. Low blood pressure levels can be found immediately postoperatively, in conditions of shock, dehydration, bleeding or heart failure, etc. All these causes of low blood pressure require immediate and accurate diagnosis and correction as they bring increased mortality [6]. Elevated blood pressure levels occur especially in patients with a history of hypertension in the context of an exaggerated postoperative catecholamine reaction, fluid overload or inadequate pain control. When they exceed certain values, beyond physiological variations, both increases and decreases in blood pressure values must be promptly corrected to prevent cerebral or cardiac events or ischemia of a recent anastomosis [7, 8]. Due to the high complexity of the measures required, it is recommended that an unstable cardiovascular patient be transferred to the intensive care unit and evaluated by a cardiologist [8].

4. Respiratory surveillance and care

The quality of respiratory function has a major impact on the patient's postoperative recovery, especially after major surgery. Immediately postoperatively, the anesthetist cleans the oropharyngeal and orotracheal cavities by suction to evacuate excessive secretions; this should be done easily so as not to increase or trigger local inflammation and spasm. Additional oxygen administration (via facemask or nasal tube) is recommended to reduce the effort of the respiratory muscles. In patients with ventilatory deficit, a high back position of 30–40 degrees can be adopted [9]; this improves respiratory dynamics and promotes the drainage of secretions [10]. For this purpose, back percussion is usually performed several times a day with the patient in sitting position, followed by respiratory toilet. The patient is encouraged to take deep breaths in order to relax and open the alveolar spaces thus reducing the ventilation "dead spaces" [9–11]. Under conditions of tracheobronchial fluid overload with excessive secretions, expectorants and mucolytics may be administered [12]; this improves drainage and reduces the effort of coughing. In such conditions, the patient is encouraged to cough in a controlled and effective manner, with the protection of the abdomen [13] (the most common site of surgery) either by gentle external pressure exerted by patient, doctor or nurse (as appropriate), or by using means of abdominal restraint like girdles. Prolonged, inefficient coughing may result in undue strain and tension on the surgical wounds, increasing the risk of evisceration or eventration. Aerosol solutions can be very useful [14] administered 2–3 times a day by nebulization for 5–10 minutes helps to "dry" or "thin" of the secretions as needed. It should be noted that postoperative pneumonia is one of the most common causes of significant morbidity and mortality after major surgery [9–11]. Prophylactic or therapeutic antibiotic therapy may not protect the patient from such a complication if excessive secretions remain undrained in the tracheobronchial tree [15]. The impact of a deficient oxygenation is systemic [16, 17], manifested at the level of the operative site (with the hypooxygenation of an anastomosis for example), at the cardiac level (decompensation of an ischemic heart disease), cerebral, etc. However supplemental oxygen should not be administered on a regular basis, but only when the oximetry drops under 90–92%, due to secondary risks of hyperoxia [18, 19]. The presence of prolonged, productive cough, especially when associated with fever and altered general condition, becomes an indication for a chest X-ray in order to capture changes responsible for the occurrence of this symptomatology and take appropriate measures [20, 21]. In this context, the findings suggest that pneumonia is a strong indication for antibiotic therapy. Irritant cough associated with sore throat and hoarseness, reported by the patient, are elements that draw attention to a digestive reflux with secondary aspiration in the airways and glottis irritation. The situation is not unusual in conditions of prolonged postoperative intestinal paresis. In such cases, the first goal is to combat gastric stasis and hyper pressure and the most rapid way is by placing a nasogastric decompression tube. If we already have a nasogastric tube in position, we need to ensure its permanent patency because the tube can be obstructed with cloths, fibrin deposits partially digested food or gastric mucosa. Otherwise, the tube becomes a reflux promoting factor by keeping the cardia open and incompetent [22]. Concurrently adopting a semi-sitting position (maintained also during sleep) to prevent or reduce reflux is an extremely useful element in combating Mendelson's syndrome (aspiration of the digestive fluid with acid content in the patient airways).

5. Surveillance of the excretory system

It is usually done by tracking the quantity and quality of urine output over a given time and more importantly in 24 hours. All patients undergoing medium and major abdominal surgery usually have a urinary catheter placed under anesthesia [23]. Catheter placement should be performed under sterile conditions, usually in preanesthetic room or on-table [24] to avoid infection, bladder injury during surgery, and to accurately monitor renal function during surgery. There are numerous causes of acute kidney injury or otherwise low urine output in the perioperative period, the risk being reported up to 5–10% in surgical patients [25]. In the immediate postoperative setting, low flow and concentrated urine indicate a good renal function but poor hydration of the patient or a state of shock due to blood loss or impaired cardiovascular function. Decreased urinary flow that occurs under conditions of proper hydration and previously normal renal function may be an indicator of fluid retention in the setting of third spacing, abdominal compartment syndrome or blood transfusions adverse reactions [10, 25]. If this event occurs within 4 to 6 days postoperatively, it is usually secondary to the development of fistular or suppurative complications at the site of surgery, alerting the surgeon and allowing a prompt diagnosis of the complication. Failure to recognize the causes and the attempt to obtain adequate diuresis can lead to overloading the patient with fluids; this impairs the function of all the systems up to acute pulmonary edema or cardiac decompensation by increased preload.

Hyperchromic urine also occurs in conditions of mechanical jaundice when the urine turns intensely yellow to brown due to the renal elimination of soluble bile pigments [26]. The presence of large amounts of urobilinogen in urine usually indicates the hemolytic or hepatocellular nature of jaundice. Hematuria is the evacuation of blood into the urine. Bleeding can be located at any level of the urinary tract from the kidneys to the urethra and usually denotes an intraoperative lesion or clotting disorder. Hematuria can be microscopic and constantly appears after pelvic or retroperitoneal surgery [27] or macroscopic - when the red color of the urine is obvious, sometimes with deposits and blood clots to the point of obvious blood (Gross hematuria). Usually, hematuria caused by minor intraoperative lesions or produced at the placement of the urethro-bladder catheter is self-limiting. Persistent hematuria requires a complete specialist diagnosis. Hemoglobinuria defines hyperchromic urine, purple to dark brown that occurs during major hemolysis after transfusion accidents [28]. Early recognition is extremely important because if undiagnosed and subsequently untreated, it can precipitate acute irreversible renal failure by blocking glomerular filtration.

The proper timing of catheter removal is debatable, numerous studies and metanalyses have addressed this question as the risk of urinary infections increases with the duration of catheterization. For abdominal surgery that does not involve the genitourinary systems or pelvic surgery it seems that the optimal timing of catheter removal is the first postoperative day [29] which in most cases coincides with the time when the patient becomes ambulatory. However, for major surgery (extensive dissection, usually for cancer) involving the pelvic organs or requiring a longer period of immobilization, the catheterization period can be extended to 3–6 days or even longer, adapted to the clinical needs [29]. For instance, whenever the bladder is sutured (after iatrogenic lesions or deliberated partial resection) the urinary catheter should be left in place for at least 10–14 days.

6. Digestive system surveillance

The digestive system is the most common surgical site in general surgery, hence the special attention paid to its care. Systematic clinical examination can provide valuable information about the patient's progress, adapting postoperative measures for an eventless and rapid recovery.

Usually forgotten or neglected, oral cavity inspection provides information about the patient's hydration level; dry oral mucosa, for instance, requires an increase in fluid intake. The presence of whitish deposits on the lingual mucosa may suggest candidiasis infection caused by prolonged antibiotic use, while red depapillated glossy mucosa suggests iron deficiency. Toileting of the oral cavity by brushing and washing with antiseptic solutions is almost as important as postoperative wound care, as germs ingested at this level colonize and contaminate the lower levels of the digestive tract accentuating dysmicrobism and promoting complications. Moreover, pathogens in the oral cavity can colonize the lung and lead to postoperative pneumonia with increased morbidity and mortality [30]. Until the patient is able to exercise basic hygiene, the task must be performed systematically by the medical personnel.

Pain therapy. Pain is one of the main factors that can delay the recovery of the operated patient. Pain delays the patient's mobilization, limits the range of motion of the diaphragm, delays the resumption of intestinal transit, and psychologically stresses the patient. Postoperative pain therapy begins during surgery, avoiding excessive traction, tension in the sutures or unjustified extensive dissections outside anatomic planes. From this point of view, laparoscopic surgery and generally mini-invasive surgery, whenever possible, brings major advantages. Also, a very important role in combating pain is the positioning of the patient in bed after surgery. The patient should be positioned as comfortably as possible, avoiding tension on the muscles around the incision areas. The movement of the patient in bed after surgery should not be forbidden; on the contrary the patient should be encouraged to adopt the position in which the pain is minimal and to change his/her position periodically. Beds with semi-rigid elastic mattresses are preferable, which can provide the patient with effective support to achieve active movements and which evenly distribute the patient's weight.

The abdomen should be examined at least twice a day. In the first 24 hours after surgery, the patient may complain of low to moderate pain in the abdomen, accentuated by active movements or coughing. The pain must be combated accordingly, in order to avoid the development of the "fear" of mobilization. Pain therapy must be adjusted to the extent of surgery and known mechanisms of pain. Multimodal postoperative analgesia appears to provide better outcomes [31]. Usually, the combination of acetaminophen with a non-steroidal anti-inflammatory drug is sufficient for most patients, but in some cases, local analgesia [32], or even patient-controlled epidural analgesia may be needed. In case of prolonged use of non-steroidal anti-inflammatory drugs (NSAID), prophylaxis of gastroduodenal disorders like erosions, hemorrhage or ulcers should be considered, especially if the patient's oral feeding has been temporarily suspended. In those cases, proton pump inhibitors and E-prostaglandin analogs seem to be the most effective, then the histamine receptors antagonists, while barrier agents are mostly useless since they do not interfere with the pathogeny of NSAID-induced ulcer. However, proton pump inhibitors are to be diverted in patients with a current or recent history of antibiotherapy, since the two conditions act synergically favouring severe *Clostridium difficile* colitis [33]. The use of major opioid analgesics is not indicated because it contributes to the accentuation of intestinal paresis and favors the accumulation of tracheobronchial secretions [34]. There are combinations of painkillers (analgesics) that combine a non-steroidal anti-inflammatory and an opioid in low concentrations where the side effects are absent or negligible. In the context of intense pain that does not yield to milder painkillers, it is recommended to place an epidural catheter to ensure the effective analgesia administration with minimal effects on the intestinal smooth muscles [35, 36].

The inspection of the abdomen helps in monitoring the degree of distension of the abdomen due to the accumulation of gases and fluids in the digestive tract lumen. This condition is mainly caused by the absence of peristalsis but also by the change of microbiome. Postoperative paresis, present after interventions involving or exposing the intestinal loops, must be actively prevented. Prevention can and should begin in the preoperative period and continue in the operating room and beyond. The very important measures are related to the optimum hydration and correction of the electrolyte imbalances. Because - Enhanced Recovery After Surgery - (ERAS) protocols have been progressively adopted, the patient is usually advised to avoid starving in the preoperative period and to have a light liquid diet in the evening, before scheduled operation. Clear fluid diet is allowed up to 2 hours preoperatively [37]. Specific medications – prokinetics - like anticholinesterases and parasympathomimetics may be prescribed in order to stimulate peristalsis [38]. Neostigmine, a synthetic anticholinesterase alkaloid, stimulates intestinal peristalsis with less extensive side effects on the cardiovascular and respiratory systems [39]. Local-acting intestinal peristaltic stimulants, such as castor oil may be administered orally or introduced through the nasogastric tube (NGT). Prolonged paresis requires the placement of an NG-tube for decompression of the digestive tract, prevention of vomiting and airway aspiration or Mendelson's syndrome. We do not usually use nasogastric decompression tube, but only in emergency surgery and just in cases associated with high fluid and gas distension or in cases with expected prolonged ileus [40].

Various methods of reducing postoperative ileus have been studied. It seems that something as simple as abdominal massage after colonic surgery can reduce the postoperative pain and help resume intestinal transit [41]. Similarly, numerous studies including a metanalysis advocate for the use of chewing gum in order to reduce the ileus period [42] but the results have been contradicted by other studies [43]. Chewing gum is adopted by the Enhanced Recovery After Surgery (ERAS) protocols as a measure that could reduce ileus [37]; we recommend its selective use whenever applicable.

Commonly used opioids such as morphine and fentanyl can prolong the postoperative ileus, by acting like agonists on mu receptors; it is recommended to reduce their use at least in the postoperative settings. In contrast, some kappa agonists like fedotozine U-50, 488H, bremazocine or asimadoline appear to reduce ileus in animal models studies but have never entered clinical practice [44, 45].

For the lower digestive tract surgery, the placement of a transanal gas tube may be used, in order to evacuate the increased pressures that may develop at this level [46]. The procedure is safe and very effective especially in low rectal anastomosis [47]. The transanal tube (TAT), usually 28–30 CH (Charrierre), is placed at the end of the procedure foiled in greased gauze and is primarily used for intraoperative leakage test. The tube is usually left in place for 48 hours or more, accordingly to the patient evolution. The TAT seems to reduce anastomotic leakage (AL), the need for re-interventions for AL, and it is proposed by some authors for the reduction of defunctioning stoma [48]. After interventions that do not involve the colon, an evacuation enema may be performed at 2–3 days postoperatively; this reduces stasis and microbial load at this level, and stimulate the resumption of normal peristalsis.

Close patient surveillance with abdominal palpation is required in order to take and adapt the appropriate postoperative measures. Palpation aims to detect possible areas of deep tenderness and infiltration in the abdomen, painful areas in which any discrete signs of peritoneal irritation draw attention to the occurrence of a complication. The jerky palpation may show flapping, a sign with great specificity for postoperative occlusive syndrome, especially when the patient has initially resumed intestinal transit. Percussion highlights diffuse tympanism during intestinal paresis, while persistent localized hypersonority in an area after hesitant resumption of intestinal transit may draw attention to a complication that may have developed at this level. Auscultating the abdomen can reveal a silent abdomen during the paretic period or vice versa- vivid noises, accompanied by whistling and crackling, an expression of the "struggle" of a loop to overcome a distal obstacle/obstruction. Anastomotic leakage is the most feared complication because it comes with significant morbidity and mortality in short but also in long term [49]. The earlier the recognition of an anastomotic leakage the better and prompter measures can be taken in order to limit or avoid major morbidity [50]. Postoperative peritonitis following an anastomotic leakage usually develops quietly and may remain undetected since the patient is on pain-killers and the peritoneal surface is less reactive after surgical aggression. CT scan can be falsely negative for anastomotic leakage in fairly large number of cases, therefore, in such cases, it is advisable to take action on first clinical signs of peritonism [51]. Measures may include various combinations of relaparotomy, percutaneous drainage, postoperative wound opening, antibiotics and complete parenteral nutrition. Earlier detection of the underlying pathology result in prompt intervention and therefore better outcomes [52]. In cases of diffuse peritonitis, relaparotomy is mandatory to remove the peritoneal contamination and try to gain control of its source. There is no ideal solution for controlling anastomotic leakage. In some cases, re-resection and anastomotic reconstruction can be an option depending on the local and general conditions. In some cases, the anastomosis may be suppressed, followed by closure of the distal end, while the proximal partner is exteriorized in a stoma. This seems to be the safest approach but it is not always feasible. In other cases, perianastomotic drainage might be enough [53], but usually a proximal diverting stoma is advisable in addition to local drainage. The decision is highly dependent on the surgeon's experience who should always thoroughly evaluate the local and general condition of the patient; it also depends on ICU level, and the local feasibility of endoscopic stenting, interventional radiology, and other interventions.

Some cases may be managed conservatively with the main purpose being to transform the leak into an isolated enterocutaneous fistula [53]. Adequate drainage of the leak results in reduction of the general and local signs of sepsis and inflammation with resuming of intestinal transit, tolerance to dietary intake and improvement of the general condition of the patient. The use of a low-pressure drainage system [54] can help organize the fistular tract, avoiding extensive contamination or digestion (by the activated intestinal enzymes) of neighboring tissues. For the success of this method, we need to ensure that the lumen of the tube remains patent and the surrounding tissues are not being sucked into the holes of the draining tube. The normal evolution of the fistula is with progressive reduction of the flow (which must be noted every 24 hours). In 5–7 days after fistular organization (clinically documented and by contrast enhanced imaging) and the reduction of the flow, we can progressively mobilize the drain by 2 cm every 2–3 days. This allows the tissues to collapse and close the fistula. Sudden reduction of a fistula flow or the early and fast suppression (in a single gesture, not progressively mobilized) of a tube that drains the leak, can result in local abscess formation or even peritonitis. Usually, the fistula closes in 2–3 weeks for the colon and 1–3 month for the small bowel but the time is variable depending on the various factors like type of surgery, age, general performance status, nutrition, level of anastomosis and partners of anastomosis quality [55], but most importantly dependent on the functional status of the bowel. If there are no anatomic (adherences or strictures for instance) or functional obstacles (residual abscess, Crohn disease, etc.) distally, the fistula closure will be faster. Insufficient drainage of the fistula or abdominal sepsis will result in persistence of local inflammation with secondary impairment of the peristaltic movements, creating a vicious circle that will delay fistula closure.

7. Postoperative wound surveillance

The postoperative wound should be closely monitored on daily basis. In the immediate postoperative period, a sterile dressing covers the wound so we may not be able to directly inspect the sutures. In the first postoperative hours soaking of the dressing [56] with blood is the main sign to look for. The presence of the blood prompts the physician to look for a source of bleeding at the superficial or deeper level and perform adequate hemostasis. In most cases, it is a low-flow bleeding from a dermal vessel that can be controlled by as simple as a local pressure dressing, placing a mesh with hydrogen peroxide, fibrin glue, or a supplementary stitch under local analgesia. This may also have psychological consequences on the patient since the psychological impact of the presence of blood in sight of the patient may induce a state of anxiety and agitation. For deeper bleedings that tend to form hematomas between the wound layers or margins, the evacuation of cloths is mandatory otherwise impairing wound healing. We should not forget that digestive surgery is a contaminated one, because of the breach of gut mucosa, and that blood is the ideal culture medium for bacteria. Therefore, leaving a dead space filled with a hematoma between the margins of the postoperative wound is equivalent with initiating a germ culture. Left in place, in the following days, the cloth will become a more or less profound abscess. At this moment, even if we drain it, the damage has happened already, and short-term morbidity as well as long-term (such as incisional hernia) increase. In order to avoid those unfavorable outcomes, the most appropriate action seems to be the immediate opening of the postoperative wound, (more or less extensive, but usually 2–4 stitches in the area of the bleeding), evacuating the hematoma under sterile conditions, lavage of the wound with antiseptic solutions, targeted hemostasis and primary closure. If there is doubt on definitive hemostasis or sterility conditions the wound can be left open, covered with sterile dressing until granulation is obtained and secondary superficial suture can be accomplished.

Sometimes under the blood-soaked dressing, we may find a diffuse bleeding, accompanied by an ecchymotic aspect of the wound edges aspects that usually indicates poor coagulation. In this context, we must not forget that the superficial operative wound is a mirror of what is happening in depth, in the operative site, and the general measures for restoring the coagulation balance must be prompt and vigorous. Of course, an ecchymosis of the postoperative wound may seem a benign and maybe minor to negligible complication requiring no action or simply a bag of ice, but if the same happens at the level of the anastomosis deep in the abdomen, anastomotic leakage becomes plausible. In this context, we immediately adjust the anticoagulation treatment, postponing or even skipping a dose until we further investigate coagulation status of the patient. As long as the anticoagulation therapy is suspended, it is advisable to use alternative methods to prevent DVT in lower limbs such as intermittent compressive therapy [57, 58] or at least compressive stockings.

In the following days, the normal surgical wound is usually uncovered, "in plain sight" or "exposed to the air". There is no reason for covering with sterile dressing since the wound is already sealed by the fibrin that is organized between the two edges. Usually, this normal wound sealing process takes 24–48 hr. in clean or clean-contaminated wounds. Even if there is no strong evidence or consensus [54, 56] on how long we should keep a sterile dressing, our current practice is to avoid dressing after 48 hr. The zonal erythema of the wound accompanied by a localized swelling, possibly centered on a slightly ecchymotic area, suggests the development of the suppurative complication. In this context, the wound must be explored with a stylus or a fine forceps inserted relatively easily in the respective area. The evacuation of a seroma or hematoma that has already turned purulent will prompt the removal of several stitches, with wide opening of the wound, followed by mechanical and antiseptic debridement [56]. Insufficient opening of the wound without adequate drainage will perpetuate the infection and allow the infection to spread to new spaces in the vicinity of the wound. In such instances a superficial infection can become profound and healing may be delayed and deficient, with wound granulomas, postoperative incisional hernias or even eviscerations. Of course, in extensive surgical site infections, local measures must be accompanied by systemic antibiotic therapy, initially with large spectrum according to the most plausible germs and then targeted when culture results become available [10, 56].

8. Postoperative drainage monitoring

Drainage is one of the fundamental means of treatment and prophylaxis in general surgery. Intraoperatively, drainage can be established in various areas of the peritoneal or pleural cavity (in the case of interventions involving the opening of the pleura), at the level of segments of the digestive tract (stomach, intestine, bile ducts) or in remaining cavities following the evacuation of pathological processes (abscesses, hydatid cysts, on the soft parts after evacuation of abscesses, hematomas, tumors, etc.).

8.1 Drainages of the peritoneal cavity

They are usually placed after medium or major and contaminated abdominal surgical interventions that open the peritoneum. That said, there is no consensus in the literature around the need for drain(s) placement after abdominal surgeries [59–61]. It is advisable to use drains only when and where they are justified. Drains are then removed in due time after they have served their purposes [62].

In the first hours after surgery, peritoneal drains usually produce small amounts of serosanguinous fluid. Pure blood drainage usually indicates a hemostasis defect that can be minor in small vessels, often secondary to clotting disorders, or major by slipping of ligatures placed on relatively large vessels. Under these conditions, it is extremely important that the drainage be interpreted in the clinical context of the patient, the association with a hemodynamic instability raising the problem of an immediate reintervention to complete the hemostasis. It is advisable to check the condition of the drain tube and especially its permeability frequently, as it can be clogged with clotted blood [63]. In this case, the tube remains unproductive, "hidden" under a clean dressing on the surface, thus providing a false sense of surgical reassurance. Unclogging of the drain tube leads to the resumption of blood flow. If the hemorrhage is still active, the drainage will be with reddish coagulable blood, drop by drop, and will be a strong indication for relaparotomy or laparoscopy [64]. In some cases, not uncommonly, the source of bleeding can be identified in the parietal trajectory of the drainage tube that intercepted a more or less important blood vessel. Local anesthesia and targeted hemostasis can save the patient from an unnecessary laparotomy. Sometimes the drainage resumes with blackish, incoagulable blood, mixed with small partially lysed cloths. This aspect of drainage, which usually persists for several days, sometimes up to weeks, indicates the progressive evacuation of a clot or a large hematoma. Particular attention must be paid in these situations to dressing maneuvers as they can lead to germ contamination and the transformation of the hematoma into an abscess.

The normal evolution of the drainage in the following days is towards the diminution and progressive clearing up. This is the optimal moment to remove the drain. When the drainage is supposed to "protect" an anastomosis we remove the tube after 5–7 days, once the anastomosis has passed the critical period and the intestinal transit is resumed [60]. The tube does not prevent anastomotic dehiscence but may avoid relaparotomy to control an anastomotic dehiscence. If the drainage is to be maintained for a longer period, it is recommended to mobilize the tubes after several days, with their dislocation from the fibrin deposits that form around, a condition for the drainage to remain effective and to prevent pressure lesions that the tube can determine on certain structures such veins, nerves, ureters, etc.

Persistence of significant drainage, over 500 mL/24 hr. (sometimes 3 L/24 hr), with serous fluid, denotes ascites production, secondary to an advanced malignancy (ovarian, peritoneal or massive hepatic metastases), liver cirrhosis or associated hypoproteinemia. Most often these conditions are suspected based on preoperative work-up and then well-documented by the intraoperative exploration. Few recent studies advise to avoid drainage in cirrhotic patients after abdominal surgery [65, 66]. If drainage is necessary, the same studies recommend discontinuing them as soon as possible. When suppressing the drain tube in these cases, a parietal restraint suture is often required to control the discharge of ascites that will otherwise persist through the parietal path of the tube. However, surgical suture dehiscence is frequent in such patients accounting between 20 and 45% [66], forced by the pressure exerted by the fluid and favored by hypoproteinemia and dysmetabolism. In those patients, we use a controlled-flow drainage tube or an abdominal decompression catheter left intraperitoneally until the wound is well healed and/or ascites production is therapeutically reduced. This management allow a controlled drainage of the ascites, in a closed system avoiding the infectious risk. Otherwise, if the tube is removed too early, intraabdominal pressure of the ascitic fluid will force the wound dehiscence and will leak uncontrollably.

After interventions involving an extended lymph node dissection, the initial drainage with serosanguinous appearance becomes sero-citrine after 2–3 days, but persistent, sometimes at flows between 50 and 300 ml / 24 h, consisting of lymph fluid rich in protein. Since there is not a consensus [67] our practice is to keep the tube in position until a significant decrease in the amount drained, otherwise there is a risk of developing lymphatic collections [68] (lymphocele), which can become secondarily infected.

Under the conditions of perianastomotic drainage, the resumption of a bloody drainage, cherry colored with low flow, sometimes gray to frank purulent with specific odor, associated or following a febrile episode is most often the sign of the onset of an anastomotic fistula. This moment usually coincides with the recurrence of the intestinal paresis, the alteration of the general condition of the patient, the increase of the digestive aspirate or vomiting. Muscle guarding may be present but the specific contracture of peritonitis is most often missing. Postoperatively, most signs of peritonism are less pronounced [69], especially in the elderly patients. Abdominal examination usually reveals localized but difficult to delineate tenderness, accompanied by a local dull pain which is accentuated on palpation. Frequently associated is the suppuration of the surgical wound that must be monitored and opened as early and as wide as needed, a unique gesture that has the ability to limit the extensive evolution in depth. Over the next few days, digestive content according to the level at which the anastomosis was performed, will be evacuated on the drain tube or directly through the surgical wound. Under the conditions of a favorable evolution, the drainage tube will be the "splint" on which an entero-cutaneous fistula forms, the inflammation then gradually decreases, the patient becomes afebrile, resumes his intestinal transit, tolerates diet, and the abdominal signs gradually subside. The development of signs of generalized peritonitis with the persistence of fever and the progressive alteration of the general condition means an insufficient drainage of the anastomotic dehiscence defining a grade C leakage [70] and forces to reintervention. Prompt diagnosis is the key for better outcomes and in this respect the CT exam seems to offer the best diagnostic chances [69]. Either conservative or interventional management is applied, in such conditions addition of antibiotherapy in curative course and a non-steroidal anti-inflammatory drug is always necessary.

8.2 The drainages of some segments of the digestive tract

The drainages of some segments of the digestive tract are generally established intraoperatively and aim at achieving temporary decompression of the organs they drain (stomach, common bile duct, etc.) As mentioned, their main role is to evacuate the secretions accumulated in the conditions of postoperative paresis and fight against intraluminal hyper pressures. The most common form is represented by the upper digestive aspiration through a nasogastric tube (NGT), in which the probe inserted trans-nasally and is conducted intraoperatively at the level of the drained segment - esophagus, stomach, duodenum, small intestine. In general, the probe is placed in the conditions of performing anastomoses or sutures at the level of these segments having as main role the protection of the suture. (*anastomotic dehiscence prophylaxis role*). The quality and quantity of the digestive aspirate must be systematically monitored and interpreted in the context of the general and local examination of the abdomen (*diagnostic tool role*). Occasionally the tube can be used to administer medications, to perform lavage or even enteral nutrition (*therapeutic role*) [71]. Congruently with literature reviews we do not systematically use the nasogastric tube [72] but only in cases with stasis, intense paresis or expected impaired temporary deglutition.

The normal evolution of the aspirate is towards "clarification" and progressive decrease in the context of the resumption of the intestinal transit and the reduction of the abdominal distension, aspects that mark the optimal moment of NGT suppression. The sudden decrease of the aspirate with the persistence or the accentuation of the distension denotes the clogging of the tube and the need to re-permeabilize it. It should not be forgotten that a significant amount of electrolytes is lost in the aspirated fluid, a loss that must be compensated by intravenous perfusion, correlated with the serum ionogram and the quality and quantity of the aspirate. Fluid loss through nasogastric tube must also be compensated by parenteral intake.

In some cases, the drainage of specific segments can be realized by tubes that are trans-parietally externalized, such as duodenostomies or jejunostomies. In the first 2–3 days postoperatively the main role of the tube is to decompress the bowel segments that they drain. The "prototype" for this use is lateral duodenostomy after total gastrectomy with "Roux en-Y" esojejunal anastomosis, in which the duodenum is partially excluded from digestive transit. After normal peristalsis resumption announced by the decreasing of the fluid output per tube over 24 hr., the drainage tube placed laterally in the duodenum can be used as a temporary feeding path [73] until the esojejunal anastomosis can support oral feeding. Although considered a "forgotten" method [73–75], the use of lateral duodenostomy gave us satisfaction (yet unpublished data), being the path that we use in order to achieve early enteral feeding, one of the main goals of ERAS protocol, especially in doubtful anastomosis or documented leakage.

External biliary drainage aims at decompressing the intra- and extrahepatic bile ducts after CBD exploration in the presence of a distal obstruction, or to obtain a controlled biliary fistula after major hydatid cyst resections or major hepatectomies [76]. The most common use is the "Kehr" drain with a "T" tube placed in the common bile duct (CBD) which will be suppressed in a controlled manner after resolving the distal obstruction or the proximal leakage. The indications for T tube decreased in the era of endoscopic retrograde colangio-pancreatography (ERCP), endoscopic drainage and stenting, etc. However, there are specific situations when the T tube remains a very good option. Usually the T tube is "guarded" by a sub-hepatic intraperitoneal drainage that in the first days after surgery will take over small amounts of bile that may leak around the T tube. In the following days the quantity and quality of bile drained by the T tube will be attentively monitored. Normal drainage should be clear bile with a flow of 3-400 ml/24 h and progressively decreasing. The persistence of a high flow clear yellow bile that sometimes can reach 1.5 l/day is a clear indication that the liver functions normally but the common bile duct is still obstructed. In those situations, the T tube becomes also a diagnostic tool, since it allows a rapid cholangiography that in most cases will clarify the diagnostic. Bile drainage containing floaters and deposits that persists for a few days raises the suspicions for intrahepatic acute cholangitis. In those cases, the T tube offers the possibility to collect seriated bile samples for bacteriology exam, culture and antibiogram, allowing thus a specific targeted antibiotherapy. In case that the drainage flow is low with a translucid uncolored fluid hepatic insufficiency should be suspected. Without becoming exhaustive in approaching an extremely complex subject, it should be mentioned that in conditions of abundant biliary drainage that persists for long periods, the imbalances induced in the body become major both by the complex loss of electrolytes, salts and bile acids but also by insufficient nutrient absorption from the digestive tract, generated by insufficient digestion. In such conditions, the reintroduction of the drained bile into the digestive tract by oral administration, via the naso-gastric tube or jejunostomy, should be considered especially in critical ill patients that do not support an internal diversion of the bile flow.

8.3 The drainage of residual cavities

The drainage of residual cavities after the evacuation of some pathological processes is generally a drainage with a long maintenance period (sometimes

1–2 month or more), time necessary for the repair processes to progressively reduce and eliminate the cavities (ex: infected hydatid cyst of the liver, pancreatic or peripancreatic abscess, etc.). The quality and quantity of drainage will be constantly monitored. Periodically the drain tube will be mobilized with dislocation of 1–2 cm in order to prevent its "anchoring" in the repair tissue, decubitus injuries on adjacent organs or structures, as well as to allow the progressive reduction of the depth of the cavity. If the drained process was a septic one, it is advisable to change periodically the drain tube since the germs tend to form biofilms on them. The profound tip of the drain will be sent for bacteriologic exam and cultures.

8.4 Drainage of the pleural cavity

Drainage of the pleural cavity is used after openings of the pleura, usually during esophageal interventions, a situation in which the drain is placed intraoperatively after re-expansion of the lung. The simplest drainage is with a transthoracic tube conducted in a half-loaded vessel with sterile saline solution, below the liquid level, to prevent pneumothorax. Mobile kits with unidirectional valves are available and considered better because they facilitate an easier and early mobilization of the patient. Normal drainage in the first days is serous, perhaps with a light serosanguinous color but with a low output, usually under 200 ml/24 h. Higher flows are reported after extended lymph node dissection (performed for esophageal carcinomas) or important bleeding [77]. The production of the bubbling phenomenon in the bottle usually denotes the existence of a "valve" through which air enters the pleural cavity - damage to the lung parenchyma or tracheobronchial-pleural fistula, another unrecognized pleural lesion (rupture), or lack of tightness of the drain tube in the parietal tract. If the intraoperative pleural lesions remain unrecognized, a situation sometimes encountered during at the esogastric junction interventions, especially in interventions for large hiatal hernias, postoperative dyspnea will require immediate clinical examination and chest X-ray which will evidence pneumothorax. In those cases, a pleural drain will be instituted under local analgesia. Pleural drainage will be removed when it becomes unproductive for gases and fluids and control X-ray will show normal pulmonary expansion, usually 5–10 days after surgery. During the removing maneuver the tube will be closed with a forceps and the parietal route will be closed with a suture and tight dressing for 24 h in order to avoid air aspiration in pleural cavity.

9. Postoperative nutrition

The postoperative diet should be strictly individualized. Current protocols recommend resuming oral feeding as early as possible [10, 37]. In conjunction with minimally invasive surgery, less aggressive anesthesia with reduced side effects, patient mobilization as early as possible, multimodal analgesia, all of which are part of the ERAS (enhanced recovery after surgery) protocol or fast track surgery.

Postoperatively, oral feeding is usually resumed progressively, starting with fluids, sometimes even from the day of surgery. Fluids can initially be administered in small amounts of "testing" of tolerance. The quantities of ingested fluids can then be increased even in the presence of the digestive tract high anastomosis [78]. In addition to the cleansing effect of the digestive tract, the dilution of toxic products and digestive enzymes, there is a proven trophic effect on the digestive mucosa, especially for glucose rich fluids, which strongly support this type of approach. The resumption of normal peristaltic and intestinal transit for gas usually marks the moment when we switch to a semi-solid diet based on vegetable purees, cheese, eggs, etc., which gradually begin to bring protein capital to the organism. Meat based products are introduced in the diet usually 2–3 days postoperatively using easy to digest white meat like fish and poultry. In the immediate postoperative period we avoid uncooked food, especially raw fruits and vegetables since their fermentative potential and fiber content that make hem harder to digest and can cause distension. After transit resuming, a banana can be daily eaten for its potassium content and then small amounts of other fruits, but always taken during the meal.

Given that in some cases the enteral diet is impractical (ex: esophageal anastomosis dehiscence) the complex products of amino acids, lipids and vitamins will be added in parenteral nutrition. Because large amounts are required it is preferably to administer them on a central venous catheter. However, it should be noted that this type of nutrition can replace the normal oral diet only for a limited time. For patients who expect a long period of oral nutrition suspension, it is preferable to perform a feeding jejunostomy [79].

10. Postoperative antibiotic therapy

Postoperative antibiotic therapy is reserved for pathologies involving extensive infections, stray patients with major interventions involving prolonged septic time, soft tissue infections, associated urinary tract infections, infectious pneumonia or another well-documented infectious syndrome.

Prolonged postoperative "so-called prophylaxis" antibiotic therapy has no justification in another context [80]. It brings major disadvantages by selecting resistant bacteria, altering the normal intestinal flora, the strain of liver and/or kidney function. In localized infections as well as in wound suppurations, the healing process starts with the appropriate drainage and not the antibiotic therapy that will be useful but to limit extensive infections and prevent dissemination. In these situations, the antibiotic therapy will be initiated according to the clinical suspected pathogen and the bacteriological profile of the nosocomial infections in the respective service, and modified according to the antibiogram after culture results are available [56].

11. Prevention of deep vein thrombosis and pulmonary thromboembolism

To this end, anticoagulant therapy is usually started preoperatively with very broad indications for interventions exceeding 30 minutes, knowing that a large number of thrombotic events in the venous system of the lower limbs begin during surgery [81]. Fractionated (or low molecular weight - LMWH) heparins as well as low dose unfractioned heparin are currently used [82]. Anticoagulant therapy is continued postoperatively for several days after the patient's usual mobilization, sometimes up to 3 weeks depending on the risks. After this period, as appropriate, anticoagulant therapy with HGMM will be replaced with oral anticoagulants - acenocoumarin derivatives, novel oral anticoagulants (NOACs) or antiaggregants. For each aspects of the anticoagulation therapy (when to start, which type, what dose, for how long, etc.) there are numerous predictive scores and tables, mostly used being the PADUA Score [83] and the Caprini Score.

In at risk patients, the calves should be inspected and palpated at least once a day. Immobilized patients are encouraged to perform active exercises in bed until complete mobilization. The appearance of a seemingly unjustified swelling or leg pain, a discrete unilateral edema of the leg, sometimes with a positive Homans sign (pain at the dorsiflexion of the foot) requires a Doppler ultrasound of the venous system of the lower limbs and the transition from prophylactic doses of anticoagulant to curative doses.

In patients with coagulation defects, with severe anemia (such as a gastrointestinal bleeding) often associated with coagulation disorders, in patients with unresectable gastrointestinal neoplasms, in polytraumatized patients with extensive hematomas at various levels or whenever heparin administration is considered risky, compressive therapy is recommended [84]. Compressive therapy can be passive, using pressure stockings, but desirable active using an intermittent compression system of the lower limbs, equipped with pneumatic cuffs that are progressively inflated and decompressed automatically, with computerized control of pressure and application times.

12. Prevention of bedsores and patient mobilization

The development of bedsores is an undesirable event that significantly influences the patient's recovery with increasing morbidity, hospitalization, medication consumption, time and resources. Elderly, deproteinized patients, diabetics, stroke patients, patients with urinary or fecal incontinence, patients with fractures or immobilized for a long time are susceptible to the development of bedsores [85]. Whenever we treat such patients, we must take into account those risk factors for an early application of bedsores prophylaxis. The most common areas affected by the development of bedsores are the sacral region, buttocks, trochanters and shoulder blades. Prophylaxis includes intermittent inflated mattresses that periodically change the pressure on the support areas, powdering of wet areas, passive mobilization for immobilized patients. They are passively transferred to alternative positions (left lateral decubitus, right lateral, dorsal, ventral) at the shortest possible time intervals (2–3 hours) after a schedule established and strictly observed. The pressure areas must be massaged to promote the opening of blood circulation in the area.

Postoperative mobilization as early as possible is an extremely important factor in the patient's recovery since it promotes the resumption of intestinal motility, reduces the risk of decubitus pneumonia and postoperative pneumonia by promoting normal respiratory dynamics, requires and stimulates the adaptation of the cardiovascular system, reduces the risk of deep vein thrombosis and thromboembolic events, prevents the appearance and development of bedsores. Thus, the patient must be passively mobilized on the edge of the bed from the first postoperative day and encouraged to repeat the maneuver several times during the day. The next day the patient will be accompanied for a few steps in the room and will later become independent at distances of 20–50 m. Of course, this mobilization program will have to be adapted to each case depending on the particularities (age, type of surgery, comorbidities, etc).

Author details

Stelian Stefanita Mogoanta[1*], Stefan Paitici[1] and Carmen Aurelia Mogoanta[2]

1 General Surgery Department, University of Medicine and Pharmacy of Craiova, Romania

2 ENT Department, University of Medicine and Pharmacy of Craiova, Romania

*Address all correspondence to: ssmogo@yahoo.com

IntechOpen

References

[1] Burke L. Postoperative fever: a normal inflammatory response or cause for concern. J Am Acad Nurse Pract. 2010 Apr;22(4):192-7. doi: 10.1111/j. 1745-7599.2010.00492.x.

[2] Hyder JA, Wakeam E, Arora V, Hevelone ND, Lipsitz SR, Nguyen LL. Investigating the "Rule of W," a mnemonic for teaching on postoperative complications. J Surg Educ. 2015 May-Jun;72(3):430-7. doi: 10.1016/j. jsurg.2014.11.004.

[3] Rosenberg-Adamsen S, Lie C, Bernhard A, Kehlet H, Rosenberg J. Effect of oxygen treatment on heart rate after abdominal surgery. Anesthesio logy. 1999 Feb;90(2):380-4. doi: 10.1097/00000542-199902000-00008.

[4] Ackland GL, Abbott TEF, Minto G, et al. Heart rate recovery and morbidity after noncardiac surgery: Planned secondary analysis of two prospective, multi-centre, blinded observational studies [published correction appears in PLoS One. 2019 Dec 5;14(12):e0226379]. PLoS One. 2019;14(8):e0221277. doi:10.1371/journal.pone.0221277

[5] Walsh SR, Tang T, Wijewardena C, Yarham SI, Boyle JR, Gaunt ME. Postoperative arrhythmias in general surgical patients. Ann R Coll Surg Engl. 2007;89(2):91-95. doi:10.1308/00358840 7X168253

[6] Lingzhong Meng, Weifeng Yu, Tianlong Wang, Lina Zhang, Paul M. Heerdt, Adrian W. Gelb, Blood Pressure Targets in Perioperative Care, Hypertension, 2018,72(4):806-817

[7] Choudhuri AH, Uppal R, Kumar M. Influence of non-surgical risk factors on anastomotic leakage after major gastrointestinal surgery: Audit from a tertiary care teaching institute. Int J Crit Illn Inj Sci. 2013;3(4):246-249. doi:10.4103/2229-5151.124117

[8] Devereaux PJ, Sessler DI. Cardiac Complications in Patients Undergoing Major Noncardiac Surgery. N Engl J Med 2015; 373:2258.

[9] Cassiday MR, Rosenkranz P, McCabe K, Rosen J, McAneny DA. I COUGH: reducing postoperative pulmonary complications with a multidisciplinary patient care program. JAMA Surg 2013;148(8):740-745.

[10] Surwit, E, Tam, T, Postoperative Care, Glob. libr. women's med., (ISSN: 1756-2228) 2008; DOI 10.3843/ GLOWM.10036Under

[11] Richard D Branson, The Scientific Basis for Postoperative Respiratory Care, Respiratory Care Nov 2013, 58 (11) 1974-1984; DOI: 10.4187/ respcare.02832

[12] Rubin BK. Secretion properties, clearance, and therapy in airway disease. Transl Respir Med. 2014;2:6. doi:10.1186/2213-0802-2-6

[13] Colucci DB, Fiore JF Jr, Paisani DM, Risso TT, Colucci M, Chiavegato LD, Faresin SM. Cough impairment and risk of postoperative pulmonary complications after open upper abdominal surgery. Respir Care. 2015 May;60(5):673-8. doi: 10.4187/ respcare.03600.

[14] Porhomayon J, Pourafkari L, El-Solh A, Nader ND. Novel therapies for perioperative respiratory complications., J Cardiovasc Thorac Res. 2017;9(3):121-126. doi:10.15171/ jcvtr.2017.21

[15] Bratzler DW, Dellinger EP, Olsen KM, Perl TM, Auwaerter PG, Bolon MK, Fish DN, Napolitano LM, Sawyer RG, Slain D, Steinberg JP, Weinstein RA; American Society of Health-System Pharmacists; Infectious Disease Society of America; Surgical

Infection Society; Society for Healthcare Epidemiology of America. Clinical practice guidelines for antimicrobial prophylaxis in surgery. Am J Health Syst Pharm. 2013 Feb 1;70(3):195-283. doi: 10.2146/ajhp120568.

[16] Karcz M, Papadakos PJ. Respiratory complications in the postanesthesia care unit: A review of pathophysiological mechanisms. Can J Respir Ther. 2013;49(4):21-29.

[17] J. F. Powell, D. K. Menon, J. G. Jones, The effects of hypoxaemia and recommendations for postoperative oxygen therapy, Anaesthesia, 1996, Volume 51, pages 769-772

[18] Suzuki, S. Oxygen administration for postoperative surgical patients: a narrative review. J intensive care 8, 79 (2020) doi.org/10.1186/ s40560-020-00498-5

[19] Hedenstierna, G., Meyhoff, C.S. Oxygen toxicity in major emergency surgery—anything new?. Intensive Care Med 45, 1802-1805 (2019). doi. org/10.1007/s00134-019-05787-8

[20] M. H. Cooper, J. N. Primrose, The value of postoperative chest radiology after major abdominal surgery, Anaesthesia, 1989, Volume 44, pages 306-309

[21] A. Miskovic, A. B. Lumb, Postoperative pulmonary complications, BJA: British Journal of Anaesthesia, Volume 118, Issue 3, March 2017, Pages 317-334, doi.org/10.1093/bja/aex002

[22] Kelkar KV. Post-operative pulmonary complications after non-cardiothoracic surgery. Indian J Anaesth. 2015;59(9):599-605. doi:10.4103/0019-5049.165857

[23] Meddings J, Skolarus TA, Fowler KE, Bernstein SJ, Dimick JB, Mann JD, Saint S. Michigan Appropriate Perioperative (MAP) criteria for urinary

catheter use in common general and orthopaedic surgeries: results obtained using the RAND/UCLA Appropriateness Method. BMJ Qual Saf. 2019 Jan;28(1):56-66. doi: 10.1136/ bmjqs-2018-008025.

[24] Nason GJ, Baig SN, Burke MJ, et al. On-table urethral catheterisation during laparoscopic appendicectomy: Is it necessary?, Can Urol Assoc J. 2015;9(1-2):55-58. doi:10.5489/cuaj.2341

[25] Chenitz KB, Lane-Fall MB. Decreased urine output and acute kidney injury in the postanesthesia care unit. Anesthesiol Clin. 2012;30(3):513-526. doi:10.1016/j.anclin.2012.07.004

[26] Beckingham IJ, Ryder SD. ABC of diseases of liver, pancreas, and biliary system. Investigation of liver and biliary disease. BMJ. 2001;322(7277):33-36. doi:10.1136/bmj.322.7277.33

[27] Esparaz AM, Pearl JA, Herts BR, LeBlanc J, Kapoor B. Iatrogenic urinary tract injuries: etiology, diagnosis, and management. Semin Intervent Radiol. 2015;32(2):195-208. doi:10.1055/s-0035-1549378

[28] Strobel E. Hemolytic Transfusion Reactions. Transfus Med Hemother. 2008;35(5):346-353. doi:10.1159/ 000154811

[29] Hendren S. Urinary catheter management. Clin Colon Rectal Surg. 2013;26(3):178-181. doi:10.1055/ s-0033-1351135

[30] Samuel J. Ford, The importance and provision of oral hygiene in surgical patients, International Journal of Surgery, Volume 6, Issue 5, 2008, Pages 418-419, ISSN 1743-9191, doi. org/10.1016/j.ijsu.2007.01.002.

[31] Wick EC, Grant MC, Wu CL. Postoperative Multimodal Analgesia Pain Management With Nonopioid Analgesics and Techniques: A Review.

JAMA Surg. 2017;152(7):691-697. doi:10.1001/jamasurg.2017.0898.

[32] Continuous local analgesia is effective in postoperative pain treatment after medium and large incisional hernia repair, MC Gherghinescu, C Copotoiu, AE Lazar, D Popa, SS Mogoanta, C Molnar, Hernia (Springer Paris), Volume 21, Issue 5, Pages 677-685, 2017)

[33] Trifan A, Stanciu C, Girleanu I, et al. Proton pump inhibitors therapy and risk of *Clostridium difficile* infection: Systematic review and meta-analysis. World J Gastroenterol. 2017;23(35): 6500-6515. doi:10.3748/wjg.v23.i35.6500

[34] Tong J. Gan, Scott B. Robinson, Gary M. Oderda, Richard Scranton, Jodie Pepin & Sonia Ramamoorthy (2015) Impact of postsurgical opioid use and ileus on economic outcomes in gastrointestinal surgeries, Current Medical Research and Opinion, 31:4, 677-686, DOI: 10.1185/03007995.2015.1005833]

[35] Popping D, Elia N, Van Aken H, et al. Impact of epidural analgesia on mortality and morbidity after surgery. Systematic review and meta-analysis of randomized controlled trials. Ann Surg 2014; 259:1056-1067.

[36] Guay J, Nishimori M, Koop S. Epidural local anesthetics versus opioid-based analgesic regimens for postoperative gastrointestinal paralysis, vomiting, and pain after abdominal surgery: a Cochrane review. Anesth Analg 2016; 123:1591-1602.

[37] Melnyk M, Casey RG, Black P, Koupparis AJ. Enhanced recovery after surgery (ERAS) protocols: Time to change practice?. Can Urol Assoc J. 2011;5(5):342-348. doi:10.5489/cuaj.11002

[38] Holte, K., Kehlet, H. Postoperative Ileus. Drugs 62, 2603-2615 (2002).

doi.org/10.2165/00003495-200262180-00004

[39] Parthasarathy G, Ravi K, Camilleri M, et al. Effect of neostigmine on gastroduodenal motility in patients with suspected gastrointestinal motility disorders. Neurogastroenterol Motil. 2015;27(12):1736-1746. doi:10.1111/nmo.12669

[40] Nelson R, Edwards S, Tse B. Prophylactic nasogastric decompression after abdominal surgery. Cochrane Database Syst Rev. 2007;2007(3): CD004929. doi:10.1002/14651858.CD004929.pub3

[41] Le Blanc-Louvry I, Costaglioli B, Boulon C, Leroi AM, Ducrotte P. Does mechanical massage of the abdominal wall after colectomy reduce postoperative pain and shorten the duration of ileus? Results of a randomized study. J Gastrointest Surg. 2002 Jan-Feb;6(1):43-9. doi: 10.1016/s1091-255x(01)00009-9.

[42] Ge W, Chen G, Ding YT. Effect of chewing gum on the postoperative recovery of gastrointestinal function. Int J Clin Exp Med. 2015;8(8): 11936-11942.

[43] Forrester DA, Doyle-Munoz J, McTigue T, D'Andrea S, Natale-Ryan A. The efficacy of gum chewing in reducing postoperative ileus: a multisite randomized controlled trial. J Wound Ostomy Continence Nurs. 2014;41:227-232.

[44] Delvaux M. Pharmacology and clinical experience with fedotozine. Expert Opin Investig Drugs. 2001 Jan;10(1):97-110. doi: 10.1517/13543784.10.1.97. PMID: 11116283.;

[45] Rivière PJ, Pascaud X, Chevalier E, Le Gallou B, Junien JL. Fedotozine reverses ileus induced by surgery or peritonitis: action at peripheral

kappa-opioid receptors. Gastroentero logy. 1993 Mar;104(3):724-31. doi: 10.1016/0016-5085(93)91007-5.

[46] Adamova Z. Transanal Tube as a Means of Prevention of Anastomotic Leakage after Rectal Cancer Surgery. Viszeralmedizin. 2014;30(6):422-426.

[47] Brandl, S. Czipin, R. Mittermair, S. Weiss, J. Pratschke, R. Kafka-Ritsch, Transanal drainage tube reduces rate and severity of anastomotic leakage in patients with colorectal anastomosis: A case controlled study, Annals of Medicine and Surgery, Volume 6,2016,Pages 12-16,ISSN 2049-0801

[48] Carboni F, Valle M, Levi Sandri GB, et al. Transanal drainage tube: alternative option to defunctioning stoma in rectal cancer surgery?. Transl Gastroenterol Hepatol. 2020;5:6. Published 2020 Jan 5. doi:10.21037/ tgh.2019.10.16

[49] Thornton M, Joshi H, Vimalachandran C, et al. Management and outcome of colorectal anastomotic leaks. Int J Color Dis. 2011;26(3):313-320. doi: 10.1007/s00384-010-1094-3.

[50] Di Cristofaro L, Ruffolo C, Pinto E, et al. Complications after surgery for colorectal cancer affect quality of life and surgeon-patient relationship. Color Dis. 2014;16(12):O407–O419. doi: 10.1111/codi.12752

[51] Kornmann VN, van Ramshorst B, Smits AB, Bollen TL, Boerma D. Beware of false-negative CT scan for anastomotic leakage after colonic surgery. Int J Colorectal Dis. 2014 Apr;29(4):445-51. doi: 10.1007/ s00384-013-1815-5

[52] Gessler, B., Eriksson, O. & Angenete, E. Diagnosis, treatment, and consequences of anastomotic leakage in colorectal surgery. Int J Colorectal Dis 32, 549-556 (2017)

[53] Creavin, B., Ryan, É.J., Kelly, M.E., Moynihan, A., Redmond, C.E., Ahern, D., Kennelly, R., Hanly, A., Martin, S.T., O'Connell, P.R., Brophy, D.P., Winter, D.C., Minimally invasive approaches to the management of anastomotic leakage following restorative rectal cancer resection. Colorectal Dis (2019), 21: 1364-1371. doi.org/10.1111/codi.14742

[54] Toon CD, Lusuku C, Ramamoorthy R, Davidson BR, Gurusamy KS. Early versus delayed dressing removal after primary closure of clean and clean-contaminated surgical wounds. Cochrane Database of Systematic Reviews 2015, Issue 9. Art. No.: CD010259. DOI: 10.1002/14651858. CD010259.pub3

[55] Pritts TA, Fischer DR, Fischer JE. Postoperative enterocutaneous fistula. In: Holzheimer RG, Mannick JA, editors. Surgical Treatment: Evidence-Based and Problem-Oriented. Munich: Zuckschwerdt; 2001. Available from: https://www.ncbi.nlm.nih.gov/books/ NBK6914/

[56] Yao K, Bae L, Yew WP. Post-operative wound management. Aust Fam Physician. 2013 Dec;42(12):867-70.

[57] Kakkos SK, Caprini JA, Geroulakos G, Nicolaides AN, Stansby G, Reddy DJ, Ntouvas I. Combined intermittent pneumatic leg compression and pharmacological prophylaxis for prevention of venous thromboembolism. Cochrane Database of Systematic Reviews 2016, Issue 9. Art. No.: CD005258. DOI: 10.1002/14651858. CD005258.pub3

[58] Lacut K, Bressollette L, Le Gal G, Etienne E, De Tinteniac A, Renault A, Rouhart F, Besson G, Garcia JF, Mottier D, Oger E; VICTORIAh (Venous Intermittent Compression and Thrombosis Occurrence Related to Intra-cerebral Acute hemorrhage) Investigators. Prevention of venous thrombosis in patients with acute

intracerebral hemorrhage. Neurology. 2005 Sep 27;65(6):865-9. doi: 10.1212/01. wnl.0000176073.80532.a2.

[59] Puleo FJ, Mishra N, Hall JF. Use of intra-abdominal drains. Clin Colon Rectal Surg. 2013;26(3):174-177. doi:10.1055/s-0033-1351134,

[60] Jesus EC, Karliczek A, Matos D, Castro AA, Atallah AN, Prophylactic anastomotic drainage for colorectal surgery., Cochrane Database Syst Rev. 2004 Oct 18; (4):CD002100.

[61] Shrikhande SV, Barreto SG, Shetty G, Suradkar K, Bodhankar YD, Shah SB, Goel M. Post-operative abdominal drainage following major upper gastrointestinal surgery: Single drain versus two drains. J Can Res Ther 2013;9:267-71

[62] Durai R, Mownah A, Ng PC. Use of drains in surgery: a review. J Perioper Pract. 2009 Jun;19(6):180-6. doi: 10.1177/175045890901900603.

[63] Yılmaz KB, Akıncı M, Şeker D, Güller M, Güneri G, Kulaçoğlu H. Factors affecting the safety of drains and catheters in surgical patients. Ulus Cerrahi Derg. 2014;30(2):90-92. Published 2014 Jun 1. doi:10.5152/UCD.2014.2564

[64] Hammond KL, Margolin DA. Surgical hemorrhage, damage control, and the abdominal compartment syndrome. Clin Colon Rectal Surg. 2006;19(4):188-194. doi:10.1055/s-2006-956439

[65] Bleszynski, M.S., Bressan, A.K., Joos, E. et al. Acute care and emergency general surgery in patients with chronic liver disease: how can we optimize perioperative care? A review of the literature. World J Emerg Surg 13, 32 (2018). doi.org/10.1186/s13017-018-0194-1

[66] Wong-Lun-Hing EM, van Woerden V, Lodewick TM,

Bemelmans MHA, Olde Damink SWM, Dejong CHC, et al. Abandoning prophylactic abdominal drainage after hepatic surgery: 10 years of no-drain policy in an enhanced recovery after surgery environment. Dig Surg. 2017;34(5):411-20.

[67] Thomson DR, Sadideen H, Furniss D. Wound drainage following groin dissection for malignant disease in adults. Cochrane Database of Systematic Reviews 2014, Issue 11. Art. No.: CD010933. DOI: 10.1002/14651858. CD010933.pub2

[68] Kim HY, Kim JW, Kim SH, Kim YT, Kim JH. An analysis of the risk factors and management of lymphocele after pelvic lymphadenectomy in patients with gynecologic malignancies. Cancer Res Treat. 2004;36(6):377-383. doi:10.4143/crt.2004.36.6.377

[69] Bader, F., Schröder, M., Kujath, P. et al. Diffuse postoperative peritonitis -value of diagnostic parameters and impact of early indication for relaparotomy. Eur J Med Res 14, 491 (2009). doi.org/10.1186/2047-783X-14-11-491

[70] Rahbari NN, Weitz J, Hohenberger W, Heald RJ, Moran B, Ulrich A, Holm T, Wong WD, Tiret E, Moriya Y, Laurberg S, den Dulk M, van de Velde C, Büchler MW. Definition and grading of anastomotic leakage following anterior resection of the rectum: a proposal by the International Study Group of Rectal Cancer. Surgery. 2010 Mar;147(3):339-51. doi: 10.1016/j.surg.2009.10.012.

[71] Tanguy M, Seguin P, Mallédant Y. Bench-to-bedside review: Routine postoperative use of the nasogastric tube - utility or futility?. Crit Care. 2007;11(1):201. doi:10.1186/cc5118

[72] Nelson R, Edwards S, Tse B. Prophylactic nasogastric decompression after abdominal surgery. Cochrane

Database Syst Rev. 2007;2007(3): CD004929. doi:10.1002/14651858. CD004929.pub3

[73] Wojciech Cwikiel Percutaneous Duodenostomy — Alternative Route for Enteral Nutrition, Acta Radiologica, 1991, 32:2, 153-154, DOI: 10.3109/02841859109177535

[74] Merhav H, Rothstein H, Simon D, Pfeffermann R. Duodenostomy revisited. Int Surg. 1988 Oct-Dec;73(4):254-6.

[75] Kutlu OC, Garcia S, Dissanaike S. The successful use of simple tube duodenostomy in large duodenal perforations from varied etiologies. Int J Surg Case Rep. 2013;4(3):279-282. doi:10.1016/j.ijscr.2012.11.025

[76] Eurich D, Henze S, Boas-Knoop S, Pratschke J, Seehofer D. T-drain reduces the incidence of biliary leakage after liver resection. Updates Surg. 2016 Dec;68(4):369-376. doi: 10.1007/s13304-016-0397-5.

[77] Lagarde SM, Omloo JM, Ubbink DT, Busch OR, Obertop H, van Lanschot JJ. Predictive factors associated with prolonged chest drain production after esophagectomy. Dis Esophagus. 2007;20(1):24-8. doi: 10.1111/j.1442-2050.2007.00639.x.

[78] Vaithiswaran V, Srinivasan K, Kadambari D. Effect of early enteral feeding after upper gastrointestinal surgery. Trop Gastroenterol. 2008 Apr-Jun;29(2):91-4.

[79] Tapia J, Murguia R, Garcia G, de los Monteros PE, Oñate E. Jejunostomy: techniques, indications, and complications. World J Surg. 1999 Jun;23(6):596-602. doi: 10.1007/pl00012353.

[80] SA Roberts, AJ Morris, Surgical antibiotic prophylaxis: more is not better, The Lancet Infectious Diseases,

2020-10-01, Volume 20, Issue 10, Pages 1110-1111

[81] Muñoz Martín, A.J., Gallardo Díaz, E., García Escobar, I. et al. SEOM clinical guideline of venous thromboembolism (VTE) and cancer (2019). Clin Transl Oncol 22, 171-186 (2020). doi.org/10.1007/s12094-019-02263-z

[82] Matar CF, Kahale LA, Hakoum MB, et al. Anticoagulation for perioperative thromboprophylaxis in people with cancer. Cochrane Database Syst Rev. 2018;7(7):CD009447. doi:10.1002/14651858.CD009447.pub3

[83] Barbar S, Noventa F, Rossetto V, Ferrari A, Brandolin B, Perlati M, De Bon E, Tormene D, Pagnan A, Prandoni P. A risk assessment model for the identification of hospitalized medical patients at risk for venous thromboembolism: the Padua Prediction Score. J Thromb Haemost. 2010 Nov;8(11):2450-7. doi: 10.1111/j.1538-7836.2010.04044.x

[84] Wille-Jørgensen P, Rasmussen MS, Andersen BR, Borly L. Heparins and mechanical methods for thromboprophylaxis in colorectal surgery. Cochrane Database Syst Rev. 2003;4:CD001217

[85] Shafipour V, Ramezanpour E, Gorji MA, Moosazadeh M. Prevalence of postoperative pressure ulcer: A systematic review and meta-analysis. Electron Physician. 2016;8(11):3170-3176. doi:10.19082/3170

Chapter 6

Special Considerations in Pediatric Abdominal Surgeries

Arwa El Rifai and Ahmad Zaghal

Abstract

Pediatric surgery, as a specialty, pertains to the diagnosis, treatment and operative management of pediatric patients with congenital as well as acquired pathologies. The physiology and functional reserve of children is different than adults and this necessitates special considerations when dealing with this subgroup of patients. This includes careful anesthesia planning, perioperative care, as well as in-depth knowledge and appreciation of anatomic variations and operative techniques.

Keywords: Pediatrics, abdominal surgery, laparoscopy

1. Introduction

> *A pearl of wisdom "Children are not small adults" [1].*

Pediatric surgery is a discipline that gradually came to light after the efforts of pioneering surgeons who dedicated their practice and refined their skills for the care of children. This sequentially provided the setting stones to establish organized training and scholarly platforms to share scientific knowledge and evidence-based practice [2].

In this chapter, we aim to highlight the peculiarities of abdominal open and minimally invasive surgery in the pediatric population with emphasis on perioperative preparation, types of incisions and wound considerations.

2. Special physiologic considerations in the pediatric patient

2.1 Anesthesia

Anesthesia in the pediatric population poses its challenges from airway management to medication prescription, however generally speaking it is well tolerated. During laparoscopy, some physiologic changes require careful management especially due to the particular patient positions as well as the pneumoperitoneum. These effects span the cardiovascular system and can manifest as bradycardia, decreased venous return, reduced cardiac output and rarely venous gas embolism. To minimize these consequences a lower insufflation pressure is recommended at 6 mmHg for infants and not above 10-12 mmHg for older children [3]. The respiratory system is also affected by the reduced diaphragmatic motion as well as the reduced lung compliance [3]. The central nervous system, the gastrointestinal system as well as coagulation can be affected as well. All these changes vary depending on patient characteristics as well as the nature and duration of the operation together with the patient position [3]. Laparoscopy, be it intraperitoneal or extraperitoneal, can have hemodynamic as well as cardiovascular effects on pediatric patients [4].

For some pathologies, such as tracheoesophageal fistula (TEF), diaphragmatic hernia and abdominal wall defects early surgical intervention might be necessary. This should not come at the expense of thorough screening of other associated anomalies that may be associated with these entities. As such, meticulous physical examination, careful cardiac evaluation with echocardiography and ultrasound examination to screen for associated congenital anomalies is key. For example, associated anomalies in TEF occur in around 50% of the patients. Therefore, the conditions within the VACTREL association should be looked for, including vertebral, anal, cardiac, renal as well as limb malformations [5]. Similarly, diaphragmatic hernia is associated with other anomalies in 40% of cases and can present with respiratory distress at birth; therefore, they require optimization of their cardiopulmonary status as well as control of pulmonary hypertension before embarking on surgical repair [6]. Lastly, congenital abdominal wall defects particularly omphalocele is associated with chromosomal, cardiac, and renal malformations [7]. In view of the possible associated anomalies and the limited physiologic reserve that pediatric patients have, some require preoperative optimization prior to the surgical intervention. For instance, evaluation and pre-operative correction of electrolytes and fluid status is crucial in cases of pyloric stenosis to avoid peri-operative ventilatory and circulatory complications [8].

Pediatric patients include neonates and infants and span up to adolescence and often the cutoff is set at 21 years of age [9]. Despite this seemingly wide continuum, the smaller the size of the patient the more restricted is the working space during surgery including laparoscopy [10]. Additionally, due to the high surface area to body mass ratio in the younger patients it is imperative to regulate intraoperative temperature to avoid the sequel of hypothermia [11].

2.2 Abdominal wall

Surgery in the pediatric age group poses a challenge due to physiologic reasons inherent to this age group. Abdominal wall elasticity is higher in this age group and can compensate for the smaller space available to operate. This is significant mainly in laparoscopic procedures whereby pneumoperitoneum is imperative for generating the space. Even though, pediatric patients have higher abdominal wall elasticity which is advantageous in laparoscopy, this is limited by the non-linearity of the relationship with intra-abdominal pressure [12]. Therefore, a balance between the added space and the optimal intra-abdominal pressure is key. Moreover, it is also important to note that the decreased thickness of the abdominal wall can pose challenges for trocar secure placement. Most laparoscopic instruments are also available in small calibers including 2-, 3- and 5-mm sizes [10].

2.3 Urethral-catheter and nasogastric tube decompression

In children, the abdominal cavity provides restricted space for operation; therefore, urinary bladder (Foley catheter) and naso-gastric decompression can deflate the bladder and stomach respectively. Moreover, depending on the surgical procedure required such as pelvic operations a urinary catheter may be required to avoid inadvertent injury [10]. As an alternative to urinary catheter insertion, in case of short operation time, some surgeons might opt for Crede's maneuver to empty the bladder [13]. This maneuver entails applying suprapubic pressure onto the bladder to decompress the bladder without instrumentation [14].

2.4 Skin preparation

An important part of preparing the patient for surgery is skin preparation with the aim of decreasing the risk of wound complications. Several solutions are available including povidone-iodine, chlorhexidine and alcohol-based solutions. In adults several studies including randomized control studies showed the superiority of using chlorhexidine-alcohol solution as compared to povidone-iodine solution with respect to prevention of wound infection [15]. In the pediatric age group, the common practice is using povidone-iodine solutions despite ample evidence on the risk especially in the neonates and premature [16]. One study assessed the transcutaneous absorption of Iodine in infants younger than 3-months and showed significant increase is plasma levels of iodine [17]. Another study demonstrated an increase in urinary excretion of iodine in infants exposed to povidone-iodine in the first months of life, this was coupled with a rise in thyrotropin as well as a decrease in thyroxine when compared to the group receiving chlorhexidine solutions [18] Comparably, the use of chlorhexidine in neonates for PICC-line care was associated with skin compromise and dermatitis [19] and some studies showed transdermal absorption [20]. There is discrepancy in evidence and the guidelines aren't clear on which type of antiseptic agent to be used [21].

2.5 Use of electrosurgical energy

The advent of electrosurgical devices was a great achievement in surgery. It allowed for precise dissection as well as hemostasis. For the neonatal and pediatric surgeons alike, it is imperative to use the lowest possible setting to get the desired effect. For monopolar devices, this includes the utilization of low-voltage continuous or blended waveforms to cut or coagulate effectively. Bipolar devices, which are considered a safer option than monopolar, use low voltage with good vessel sealing effects with minimal collateral tissue damage [22].

3. Open surgery in the pediatric patient

When evaluating an infant or a child, timely diagnosis and treatment are essential in view of the limited physiologic reserve these patients have. The most common abdominal emergencies in pediatrics are acute appendicitis, symptomatic hernia, intussusception as well as congenital anomalies such as atresia and malrotation [23].

3.1 Access for open surgery

Whenever planning an operation, special considerations need to be entertained for choosing the type of incision. This often takes into account the surgical pathology, the contamination status as well as the patient's anatomy, the most commonly used incision in the pediatric age group is the transverse laparotomy incision.

3.2 Access for redo surgery

Reoperations, planned or unplanned, can pose significant morbidity in adults as well as in children. Several indications for reoperation arise in the pediatric age group, these include wound complications, bleeding as well as intra-abdominal infections [24]. One of the important considerations in reoperations is incision planning since adhesions are likely to form and bowel loops might adhere to the wound site. This may constitute an increased risk of iatrogenic injuries while trying to gain access to the abdominal cavity [25]. One way to avoid this is choosing a virgin area for the incision.

3.3 Laparotomy incisions

In infants, unlike adults, a supraumbilical transverse incision provides exposure to the whole abdomen. On the other hand, the midline laparotomy incision is less commonly used in children as compared to adults. It is found to be associated with higher risk of dehiscence in comparison to the transverse laparotomy incision [26]. Depending on the surgical pathology other incision types can be used.

3.4 Subcostal incisions

A subcostal incision, also known as Kocher incision can be performed when access to the right and left upper quadrants is needed. As such a left subcostal incision can provide access to the spleen, diaphragm and esophagus. A right subcostal incision can provide access of the biliary tree in major hepatobiliary operations. The incision is generally started in the midline at the subxiphoid area and extended laterally parallel to the costal margin. The incision can be extended to gain better exposure bilaterally as a rooftop modification. Another modification that can be used in liver transplant surgery is the Mercedes-Benz modification. It entails fashioning the subcostal incisions lower than the standard unilateral subcostal incision with an extension in the midline towards the xyphoid process [27].

3.5 Trans-umbilical incision

Another less invasive access to the peritoneal cavity in children utilizes the trans-umbilical route and utilizes the advantageous abdominal wall elasticity to have a large operating field. It is performed by incising circumferentially around the umbilicus completely or partially and then incising the fascia in the midline and accessing the peritoneum guided by the site of the pathology [28]. The circum-umbilical access in children was first utilized to perform a pyloromyotomy in 1986 [29] and since then it has been used for several operations such as hypertrophic pyloric stenosis and intestinal atresia repair [28] This access technique is gaining popularity in older children for operations such as Meckel's diverticulum and ovarian cysts with comparable operative time and good cosmesis [30]. A wound protector can be utilized to stretch the wound further and allow exteriorization of the specimen as needed. Moreover, the incision can be extended to form an "Omega sign" and gain wider access if deemed necessary. Also, a variation to the incision can be done by performing it at the outer umbilical fold [30]. As compared to the traditional transverse incision one study by Suri et al. reported comparable operative times, use of narcotics as well as length of hospital stay and wound infection rate. However, they noted a higher hernia rate than the transverse incision group but not requiring operative intervention for resolution [31]. During umbilical access in the neonates, it is necessary to carefully ligate any urachal remnant, umbilical vessels or vitelline duct remnants [32].

3.6 Other incisions

Despite the decreased popularity of the open approach for acute appendicitis, it is still used in certain cases of complicated appendicitis, lack of laparoscopic equipment and expertise. The open approach using a McBurney/Gridiron incision which is an oblique right lower quadrant incision or a more transverse Lanz incision in the same quadrant [33].

Another common incision used in pediatric surgery is the Pfannenstiel incision. It provides a wide surgical field and good cosmetic result. It has been used for repair of inguinal hernia in emergency setting [34] as well as in urologic operations [35]. Another lower abdominal incision, the concealed arch incision, has been used in pediatric urologic surgery. It involves an incision, mainly in females, fashioned on the inner aspect of the labia majora bilaterally with care taken to avoid the clitoris. This incision was shown to provide similar exposure as the traditional Pfannesntiel incision [36].

Another commonly used incisions are those needed to access the gastrointestinal tract either for decompression or for diversion of fecal stream. In children most commonly a sigmoid or transverse colostomy are most commonly used. Stomas are fashioned away from the laparotomy incision (if any) and are brought through the rectus muscle.

Depending on the segment of bowel chosen a right or left lower quadrant incision is used or an upper quadrant site for a transverse colostomy [37].

4. Laparoscopic surgery in the pediatric patient

Laparoscopic surgery has gained popularity ever since it was first described by Kelling in 1923 [38]. It includes working in the peritoneal cavity as well as the retroperitoneal space covering a myriad of procedures such as gastrointestinal and urologic procedures. However, the abdominal cavity in children and neonates is much smaller posing some technical challenges as well as a steep learning curve for most pediatric laparoscopic procedures [10]. The most common procedures performed for children are cholecystectomy, appendectomy and fundoplication. Some of the complications associated with these surgeries include wound infection, abscess formation as well as obstruction. These complications are noted to occur at a lower rate when compared to open surgery [39].

4.1 Access for laparoscopy

Several techniques are available to gain access to the peritoneal cavity for the purpose of performing a laparoscopic or a robotic procedure. Open access method is one technique of gaining entry to the peritoneal cavity, it entails making an incision usually for the camera port and then incising the peritoneum under direct vision. This is a very safe method and reduces the risk of inadvertent injury to the abdominal viscera during entry. Another method of entry to the abdominal cavity and establishing pneumoperitoneum is via the Veress needle. It utilizes a special needle that penetrates through the abdominal wall and alerts the surgeon by transmitting two haptic pops indicating successful entry. Moreover, correct placement can be tested by aspiration using a syringe with no blood or enteric fluid return. Lastly, direct access can be used, in this technique a transparent trocar is placed directly over the incision and using the scope penetration of the abdominal wall layers is done under vision. Regardless of the access method, the risk of inadvertent injury decreases with operator experience [10].

4.2 Single-incision

As part of the thrive for minimally invasive approaches to surgery, the advent of single-incision operations came about. By definition, it is surgery performed using one incision through which access to the abdomen, chest or retroperitoneum will be provided. The first pediatric single-incision operation was an appendectomy done in 1998 [40]. Since then, several operations have been attempted using this approach. Besides the most commonly performed appendectomy, Inguinal hernia repairs were second in frequency followed by cholecystectomy and varicocelectomy [41]. For single-port operation in children, the umbilicus is of small caliber and thus restricts instrumentation and specimen exteriorization. The Benz incision, an inverted Y-shaped incision, through the umbilicus has been reported as a means to overcome this [42].

4.3 Robotic surgery

Some of the challenges faced in laparoscopic surgery can be overcome by using the robotic platforms. Robotic surgery allows higher precision and ease of instrumentation with 360-degree hand movements while providing a three-dimensional view [10].

5. Closure techniques and use of drains

Abdominal closure techniques encompass mass or layered closure with variable use of absorbable versus non-absorbable suture material, monofilament versus polyfilament and continuous versus interrupted patterns [43]. The literature is scarce on comparing each technique of closure in the pediatric age group. A Cochrane review that looked at studies in adults and children regarding wound closure concluded absorbable suture material resulted in less risk of fistulization. Moreover, it showed no superiority of interrupted versus continuous closure techniques with respect to hernia formation. Lastly, the use of monofilament sutures was associated with reduced hernia risk [44]. Evidence regarding the long-term effect of abdominal wall closure technique is scarce and stems from literature with prolonged follow up until adulthood in patients undergoing surgery for congenital abdominal wall defects in infancy. One study reported on the need for reoperation later in life in up to 22% of the patients due to occurrence of hernias or sequelae of atresia [45]. Another study reported that adult patients who had congenital abdominal wall defects repaired in childhood showed comparable quality of life as the general population [46]. The common practice nowadays is to use absorbable sutures to close abdominal wall defects as well as surgical incisions including laparotomies [44]. These sutures will dissolve before a significant abdominal wall growth is noted and hence unlikely to affect or retard growth.

5.1 Use of drains

Drain insertion after surgery is debatable with the theoretical benefit of clearance of residual infection, debris and as a window to hemostasis. One of the most common operations where drains are used is perforated appendicitis. In these cases, a Jackson-Pratt (JP) drain is commonly used which utilizes a negative pressure closed system to clear fluid. However, evidence against the use of JP drains is accumulating with evidence showing increased postoperative complications including abscess formation, and small bowel obstruction [47]. Another study failed to show decrease in intra-abdominal abscess formation with the use of Blake drains in perforated appendicitis [48]. If a drain was placed after perforated appendicitis, the timing of removal is dictated by the output volume and character. It is generally considered optimal to remove drains once output is clear and less than 20 ml/day [49]. Another classic indication for drain insertion is after Roux-en-Y hepatojejunostomy in choledochal cyst operations, However, with the advent of laparoscopy the use of drains after this operation is reserved for a particular subset of patients with significant inflammation at the operative field, perforated biliary peritonitis and a cyst that is majorly embedded within the pancreatic parenchyma [50].

Yet there remains a role for drains in certain clinical scenarios. This includes placement of Penrose drain in a subcutaneous abscess cavity after adequate drainage and debridement of infected wounds and abscesses. Often these drains are removed once the drainage from the cavity is minimal and surrounding soft tissue infection has resolved [51]. Moreover, there is a potential role for peritoneal drainage as a definitive measure in necrotizing enterocolitis (NEC) with perforation with or without laparotomy as clinically indicated in the course of follow up [52].

6. Wound considerations

Wound complications can pose a serious postoperative morbidity on surgical patients including children. The incidence ranges from 0.4 [26] to 1.2% [53] however it has a high mortality rate that can range from 8% [26] up to 34% in cases of evisceration [54]. Several risk factors have been reported including vertical incisions namely in children younger than one year of age [26]. Other independent risk factors included age less than one-year with an odds ratio of 9.5, wound infection OR 3.7, median incision OR 2.9 and emergency surgery 2.8 [55].

7. Conclusion

Despite the similarities in surgical principles between adult and pediatric surgery it is imperative to appreciate the differences that remain. With this in mind, surgical pathologies in the pediatric age group remain the most diverse and intriguing yet challenging cases.

Conflict of interest

The authors declare no conflict of interest.

Author details

Arwa El Rifai and Ahmad Zaghal*
Department of Surgery, American University of Beirut Medical Center,
Beirut, Lebanon

*Address all correspondence to: az22@aub.edu.lb

IntechOpen

References

[1] Gillis J, Loughlan P. Not just small adults: the metaphors of paediatrics. Arch Dis Child. 2007: 92(11):946-947. DOI: 10.1136/adc.2007.121087

[2] Ziegler M, Azizkhan R, Allmen D, Weber T. Chapter 1: History of Pediatric Surgery. Operative Pediatric Surgery, 2nd ed, McGraw-Hill; 2014

[3] Gupta R, Singh S. Challenges in Paediatric Laparoscopic Surgeries. Indian J Anaesth. 2009: 53(5):560-566. PMCID: PMC2900088, PMID: 20640106

[4] Halachmi S, El-Ghoneimi A, Bissonnette B. Hemodynamic and Respiratory Effect of Pediatric Urological Laparoscopic Surgery: A Retrospective Study. The Journal of Urology. 2003:170:1651-1654. DOI: 10.1097/01.ju.0000084146.25552.9c

[5] De Jong E, Felix J, De Klein A, Tibboel D. Etiology of Esophageal Atresia and Tracheoesophageal Fistula: "Mind the Gap". Curr Gastroenterol Rep (2010) 12:215-222 DOI: 10.1007/s11894-010-0108-1

[6] Wynn J, Yu L, Chung W. Genetic causes of congenital diaphragmatic hernia. Semin Fetal Neonatal Med. 2014 December; 19(6): 324-330. DOI:10.1016/j.siny.2014.09.003

[7] Mann S, Blinman T, Wilson R. Prenatal and postnatal management of omphalocele. Prenat Diagn 2008; 28: 626-632. DOI: 10.1002/pd.2008

[8] Kamata M, Cartabuke R, Tobias J. Perioperative care of infants with pyloric stenosis. doi:10.1111/pan.12792. DOI:10.1111/pan.12792

[9] Hardin A, Hackell J. Age Limit of Pediatrics. Pediatrics. 2017: 140(3): e20172151. DOI: 10.1542/peds.2017-2151

[10] Tomaszewski J, Casella D. Pediatric Laparoscopic and Robot-Assisted Laparoscopic Surgery: Technical Considerations. Journal of Endourology. 2012: 26(6):602-613. DOI: https://doi.org/10.1089/end.2011.0252

[11] Bindu B, Bindra A, Rath G. Temperature management under general anesthesia: Compulsion or option. J Anaesthesiol Clin Pharmacol. 2017: 33(3):306-316. DOI: 10.4103/joacp.JOACP_334_16

[12] Zhou R, Cao H, Gao Q. Abdominal Wall Elasticity of Children during Pneumoperitoneum. Journal of Pediatric Surgery. 2020:55(4):742-746. DOI: 10.1016/j.jpedsurg.2019.05.025

[13] Lobe T. Chapter 36: Pediatric Laparoscopy: General Considerations. Page 387. C. E. H. Scott-Conner (ed.), The SAGES Manual Society of American Gastrointestinal Endoscopic Surgeons 1999

[14] Barbalia G, Klauber G, Blaivas J. Critical Evaluation Of The Crede Maneuver: A Urodynamic Study Of 207 Patients. The Journal of Urology. Volume 130, Issue 4, October 1983, Pages 720-723. https://doi.org/10.1016/S0022-5347(17)51423-8

[15] Darouiche R, Wall M, Itani K. Chlorhexidine-Alcohol versus Povidone-Iodine for Surgical-Site Antisepsis. N Engl J Med. 2010: 362(1):18-26. DOI: 10.1056/NEJMoa0810988

[16] Ng A, Jackson C, Kazmierski M. Evaluation of Antiseptic Use in Pediatric Surgical Units in the United Kingdom—Where Is the Evidence Base?. European Journal of Pediatric Surgery. 2016 Aug;26(4):309-315. DOI: 10.1055/s-0035-1559883

[17] Mitchell I, Pollock J, Jamieson M, Fitzpatrick K, Logan R. Transcutaneous

iodine absorption in infants undergoing cardiac operation. Ann Thorac Surg. 1991: 52(5):1138-1140. DOI: 10.1016/0003-4975(91)91295-7

[18] Smerdely P, Lim A, Boyages S. Topical iodine-containing antiseptics and neonatal hypothyroidism in very-low-birthweight infants. Lancet. 1989: 2(8664):661-664. DOI: 10.1016/s0140-6736(89)90903-3

[19] Visscher M, deCastro M, Combs L. Effect of chlorhexidine gluconate on the skin integrity at PICC line sites. J Perinatol. 2009: 29(12):802-807. DOI: 10.1038/jp.2009.116

[20] Owen J, Ellis SH, McAinsh J. Absorption of chlorhexidine from the intact skin of newborn infants. Arch Dis Child. 1979: 54(5):379-383. DOI: 10.1136/adc.54.5.379

[21] Loveday H, Wilson J, Pratt R. epic3: National Evidence-Based Guidelines for Preventing Healthcare-Associated Infections in NHS Hospitals in England. J Hosp Infect. 2014 Jan; 86: S1–S70. DOI: 10.1016/S0195-6701(13)60012-2

[22] Sinha S, Dhua A. Energy Sources in Neonatal Surgery: Principles and Practice. Journal of Neonatal Surgery 2014;3(2):17. PMCID: PMC4420325. PMID: 26023488

[23] Firomsa T, Teferra M, Tadesse A. Trends and Outcomes of Emergency Pediatric Surgical Admissions from a Tertiary Hospital in Ethiopia. Ethiop J Health Sci. 2018:28 (3):251-258. DOI: 10.4314/ejhs.v28i3.2

[24] Li A, Zhu H, Zhou H, Liu J, Deng Y, Liu Q, Guo C. Unplanned surgical reoperations as a quality indicator in pediatric tertiary general surgical specialties: Associated risk factors and hospitalization, a retrospective case–control analysis. Medicine 2020;99:19

(e19982). http://dx.doi.org/10.1097/MD.0000000000019982

[25] Coleman M, Mclain A, Moran B. Impact of Previous Surgery on Time Taken for Incision and Division of Adhesions During Laparotomy. Dis Colon Rectum 2000;43:1297-1299. DOI: 10.1007/BF02237441

[26] Waldhausen J, Davies L. Pediatric Postoperative Abdominal Wound Dehiscence: Transverse Versus Vertical Incisions. J Am Coll Surg. 2000 Jun;190(6):688-691. DOI: 10.1016/s1072-7515(00)00284-2

[27] Bradnock Tm Carachi R. 2013) A10 Subcostal and Rooftop Incisions. In: Carachi R., Agarwala S., Bradnock T.J., Lim Tan H., Cascio S. (eds) Basic Techniques in Pediatric Surgery. Springer, Berlin, Heidelberg. https://doi.org/10.1007/978-3-642-20641-2_10

[28] Elhalaby E, Hassan H, Hashish M, Hashish A. The versatility of the transumbilical approach for laparotomy in infants. Annals of Pediatric Surgery. 2015:11(1):1-6. DOI: 10.1097/01.XPS.0000459975.88923.a6

[29] Tan K, Bianchi A. Circumumbilical incision for pyloromyotom. Br J Surg. 1986:73(5):399. DOI: 10.1002/bjs.1800730529

[30] Tsuji Y, Maeda K, Ono S, Yanagisawa S. A new paradigm of scarless abdominal surgery in children: Transumbilical minimal incision surgery. Journal of Pediatric Surgery. 2014:49:1605-1609. DOI: 10.1016/j.jpedsurg.2014.06.009

[31] Suri M, Langer J. A comparison of circumumbilical and transverse abdominal incisions for neonatal abdominal surgery. Journal of Pediatric Surgery. 2011: 46(6):1076-1080. DOI: 10.1016/j.jpedsurg.2011.03.032

[32] Hegazy A. Anatomy and embryology of umbilicus in newborns:

a review and clinical correlations. Frontiers of Medicine. 2016:10(3):271-277. DOI: 10.1007/s11684-016-0457-8

[33] Khirallah M, Eldesouki N, Elzanaty A, Ismail K, Arafa M. Laparoscopic versus open appendectomy in children with complicated appendicitis. Ann Pediatr Surg 13:17-20. DOI: 10.1097/01. XPS.0000496987.42542.dd

[34] Koga H, Yamataka A, Ohshiro K, Okada Y. Pfannenstiel Incision for Incarcerated Inguinal Hernia in Neonates. Journal of Pediatric Surgery volume 38:8, E16E18. DOI:https://doi. org/10.1016/S0022-3468(03)00293-8

[35] Kim C, Docimo S. Use of Laparoscopy in Pediatric Urology. Rev Urol. 2005;7(4):215-223

[36] Snow B. Journal of Pediatric Urology (2015) xx, 1e2, Journal of Pediatric Urology (2015) xx, 1e2. http://dx.doi.org/10.1016/j. jpurol.2015.05.021

[37] Minkes R, Grewal H. Stomas of the Small and Large Intestine in Children Treatment & Management [Internet]. 2019. Available from: https://emedicine. medscape.com/article/939455-treatment#d1 [Accessed: 2021-01-22]

[38] Litynski G. Laparoscopy - The Early Attempts: Spotlighting Georg Kelling and Hans Christian Jacobaeus. JSLS. 1997:1(1):83-85. PMID: 9876654, PMCID: PMC3015224

[39] Billingham M, Basterfield S. Pediatric Surgical Technique: Laparoscopic or Open Approach? A systematic Review and Meta-Analysis. Eur J Pediatr Surg. 2010:20(2):73-77. DOI: 10.1055/s-0029-1241871

[40] Esposito C. One-trocar appendectomy in pediatric surgery. Surg Endosc. 1998:12(2):177-178. DOI: 10.1007/s004649900624

[41] Saldana L, Targarona E. Single-Incision Pediatric Endosurgery: A Systematic Review. Journal of Laparoendoscopic & Advanced Surgical Techniques. 2013 May;23(5):467-480. DOI: 10.1089/lap.2012.0467

[42] Amano H, Uchinda H, Kawashima H. The Umbilical Benz Incision for Reduced Port Surgery in Pediatric Patients. JSLS. 2015;19(1):e2014.00238. DOI: 10.4293/ JSLS.2014.00238

[43] Khan S, Saleem M, Talat N. Wound dehiscence with continuous versus interrupted mass closure of transverse incisions in children with absorbable suture: a randomized controlled trial. World Jnl Ped Surgery. 2019;2:e000016. DOI:10.1136/wjps-2018-000016

[44] Patel S, Paskar D, Nelson R. Closure methods for laparotomy incisions for preventing incisional hernias and other wound complications. Cochrane Database of Systematic Reviews. 2017 Nov; 2017(11): CD005661. DOI: 10.1002/14651858.CD005661.pub2

[45] Tunell W, Puffinbarger N, Tuggle D, Taylor D, Mantor P. Abdominal Wall Defects in Infants Survival and Implications for Adult Life. Ann Surg. 1995 May; 221(5): 525-530. DOI: 10.1097/00000658-199505000-00010

[46] Koivusalo A, Lindahl H, Rintala R. Morbidity and quality of life in adult patients with a congenital abdominal wall defect: a questionnaire survey. J Pediatr Surg. 2002 Nov;37(11):1594-1601. doi: 10.1053/jpsu.2002.36191

[47] Song R, Jung K. Drain insertion after appendectomy in children with perforated appendicitis based on a single-center experience. Ann Surg Treat Res 2015;88(6):341-344. http:// dx.doi.org/10.4174/astr.2015.88.6.341

[48] Ferguson D, Anderson K, Arshad S, et al., Prophylactic intraabdominal

drains do not confer benefit in pediatric perforated appendicitis: Results from a quality improvement initiative. Journal of Pediatric Surgery, In Press. https://doi.org/10.1016/j.jpedsurg.2020.06.031.

[49] Eysenbach L, Caty M, Christison-Lagay E, Cowles R. Outcomes following adoption of a standardized protocol for abscess drain management in pediatric appendicitis. Journal of Pediatric Surgery 56 (2021) 43-46. https://doi.org/10.1016/j.jpedsurg.2020.09.050

[50] Diao M, Li L, Cheng W. To drain or not to drain in Roux-en-Y hepatojejunostomy for children with choledochal cysts in the laparoscopic era: a prospective randomized study. Journal of Pediatric Surgery (2012) 47, 1485-1489. DOI:10.1016/j.jpedsurg.2011.10.066

[51] Ladd A, Levy M, Quilty J. Minimally invasive technique in treatment of complex, subcutaneous abscesses in children. Journal of Pediatric Surgery (2010) 45, 1562-1566. DOI:10.1016/j.jpedsurg.2010.03.025

[52] Downward C, Renaud E, Peter S, Abdullah F. Treatment of necrotizing enterocolitis: an American Pediatric Surgical Association Outcomes and Clinical Trials Committee systematic review. Journal of Pediatric Surgery (2012) 47, 2111-2122. http://dx.doi.org/10.1016/j.jpedsurg.2012.08.011)

[53] Gruessner R, Pistor G, Kotei DN. Relaparotomie im Kindesalter [Relaparotomy in childhood], Langenbecks Arch Chir, 1986: 367(3):167-180. DOI: 10.1007/BF01258935

[54] Cığdem M, Onen A, Otcu S, Duran H. Postoperative abdominal evisceration in children: possible risk factors. Pediatr Surg Int (2006) 22:677-680 DOI 10.1007/s00383-006-1722-8

[55] Ramshorst G, Salu N, Bax N. Risk Factors for Abdominal Wound Dehiscence in Children: A Case-Control Study. World J Surg. 2009 Jul;33(7):1509-1513. DOI: 10.1007/s00268-009-0058-7